Mental Health: Global Policies and Human Rights

Edited by

PETER MORRALL PhD, MSc, BA(HONS), PGCE, RN
Senior Lecturer in Health and Sociology, University of Leeds, UK

and

MIKE HAZELTON PhD, MA, BA, FANZCMHN, RN
Professor of Mental Health Nursing, University of Newcastle
and Hunter Mental Health Service, Australia

W
WHURR PUBLISHERS
ONDON AND PHILADELPHIA

© 2004 Whurr Publishers Ltd
First published 2004
by Whurr Publishers Ltd
19b Compton Terrace
London N1 2UN, England and
325 Chestnut Street, Philadelphia PA 19106, USA

Reprinted 2005

British Library Cataloguing in Publication Data

A catalogue record for this book
is available from the British Library.

ISBN 1 86156 388 4

Typeset by Adrian McLaughlin, a@microguides.net
Printed and bound in the UK by Athenæum Press Limited, Gateshead, Tyne & Wear

Contents

Contributors

Dr Domingos Nascimento Alves (Brazil) Neurologist; specialist in social psychiatry and public health; President of the Instituto Franco Basaglia in Rio de Janeiro, Brazil. Former National Co-ordinator of Mental Health at the Brazilian Ministry of Health; activist for the transformation of national reality in the field of mental health in Brazil.

Associate Professor Lorenzo Burti (Italy) Associate Professor of Psychiatry, Department of Medicine and Public Health, Section of Psychiatry, University of Verona, Italy; Associate Clinical Director, South-Verona Community Mental Health Service; Founding President, Italian Association for Psychosocial Rehabilitation; author/co-author of more than 130 scientific publications; co-author of three books on community psychiatry and rehabilitation.

Professor Michael Clinton (Australia) Dean (Organisational Management), Division of Health Sciences, Curtin University of Technology, Perth, Western Australia; publisher of numerous books, book chapters and articles in national and international journals on nursing, mental health nursing, and mental health policy; consultant to the International Council of Nurses; former President of the Australian and New Zealand College of Mental Health Nurses.

Dr Viviana Galli (China) Psychiatrist; researcher and teacher at University of Cincinnati Department of Psychiatry, College of Medicine, University of Cincinnati, Ohio, USA; Medical Director in charge of the management and clinical supervision of an out-patient substance abuse programme; training officer in charge of psychiatric continuing education in a military field unit; author of numerous articles on psychiatric medicine, and human rights abuse of Falun Gong members in China.

Professor Mike Hazelton (Australia) Professor of Mental Health Nursing, University of Newcastle and Hunter Mental Health Service, New South Wales, Australia; sociologist; Editor of the *International Journal of Mental Health Nursing*; author/co-author of over 40 book chapters and journal articles, published in the nursing, sociology and medical literature.

Victor Igreja (Mozambique) Psychologist, pedagogue and medical anthropologist; main trauma researcher in the former war zones of central Mozambique, working with the Non-Governmental Organisation *Associação Esperança para Todos – AEPATO* [Hope for Everyone]; involved since 1996 in a mental health project on the long-term effects of the war; trying to develop a community-based model encompassing traditional and religious healing practices, the customary justice system, and the agricultural cycle to respond to the physical and mental health needs of war survivors; affiliated researcher (WOTRO) at Leiden University Medical Centre, Department of Culture, Health and Illness, and the African Study Centre (Leiden, The Netherlands).

Dr Sunny Yang Lu (China) Psychiatrist; Adjunct Clinical Assistant Professor in the Department of Psychiatry, College of Medicine, University of Cincinnati, Ohio, USA; born in Beijing, experienced communist China's 'cultural revolution' growing up as a young woman; author of numerous articles on neurological medicine, and human rights abuse of Falun Gong members in China.

Dr Peter Morrall (UK) Senior Lecturer in Health and Sociology, School of Health Care Studies, University of Leeds, UK; author of numerous articles and book chapters on mental health, and three books – *Madness and Murder* (2000, London: Whurr), *Mental Health Nursing and Social Control* (1998, London: Whurr), and *Sociology and Nursing* (2001, London: Routledge).

Professor R. Srinivasa Murthy (India) Professor of Psychiatry, National Institute of Mental Health and Neurosciences, Bangalore, India; member of the World Health Organization Expert Mental Health Advisory Committee; author of over 200 articles in national and international journals, and international monographs; member of the Education Committee of the World Psychiatric Association; Chief Editor of *World Health Report 2001: Mental Health: New Understanding, New Hope*; pioneered and/or assisted in the formulation and evaluation of mental health programmes in India, Nepal, Yemen, Bhutan, Pakistan, Iran, Sri Lanka, and Afghanistan.

Professor Ahmed Okasha (Egypt) President of World Psychiatric Association; Director the World Health Organization Collaborating Centre for Training and Research in Mental Health, Institute of Psychiatry, Ain Shams University, Cairo, Egypt; author/co-author of more than 250 original articles in national and international journals, and a number of books in Arabic and English about mental health and psychiatry.

Dr Yuri S. Savenko (Russia) President of the Independent Psychiatric Association of Russia; Editor-in-Chief of the Independent Psychiatric Journal; member of the Expert Council, Russian Federation Ombudsman; Chairman of the Psychiatry and Human Rights section of the Expert Council, Russian Federation Ombudsman; member of the Supreme Soviet Commission for Preparing the Draft on Psychiatric Care (1990–1991); member of the Russian State Duma Commission for Preparing the Draft on Psychiatric Care (1991–1992); member of the Russian Health Ministry's Commission on Preparing, Changing and Supplements to the Law on Psychiatric Care (2000–2001).

Professor Shirley A. Smoyak (USA) Planning, psychiatric nurse, and health care sociologist, Bloustein School of Planning and Public Policy, Department of Urban Studies and Community Health, Rutgers State University, New Jersey, USA; Editor of the *Journal of Psychosocial Nursing and Mental Health Services*; author of several books, many refereed journal articles, chapters, monographs and videotapes.

Dr Willians Valentini (Brazil) Psychiatrist and Superintendent at Serviço de Saúde Dr Cândido Ferreira, Sousas, Campinas, São Paulo, Brazil since 1991; author of numerous publications on psychosocial rehabilitation and management in mental health services; consultant for the National Co-ordination of Mental Health of the Ministry of Health in Brazil since 1992. Consultant for the World Health Organization in Barbados, West Indies, in 1995. National Secretary for the World Association for Psychosocial Rehabilitation in 1998, 1999 and 2000 in Brazil; former consultant for the World Health Organization in Barbados, West Indies, and Mozambique.

Introduction

PETER MORRALL AND MIKE HAZELTON

Mental health has become a major global problem. It affects 450 million people and one in four of us will suffer from mental ill-health at some time in our lives (WHO, 2001).

Throughout both the developed and developing regions of the world the treatment and care of the mentally disordered, the prevention of mental health problems, and the improvement of the mental health status of all citizens, have entered the political domain at national and international levels. Issues concerning mental health have been raised substantially in the consciousness of politicians, the media, and the public. Moreover, the 'burden' of mental disorder is regarded not just as a – if not *the* – principal cause of human misery, but as a significant impediment to social and economic growth. Measurement of the years of potential life lost and the years of productive life lost (disability-adjusted life years – DALY) through mental ill-health could reach 15% of all diseases and deaths globally by 2020 (WHO, 1999).

The effects on mental health of globalization, mass electronic communication, vast population shifts and the creation of large collections of refugees, growing health and social divides, totalitarianism, fundamentalism, warfare within and between countries, the economic advancement of China, new configurations of civil strife as the result of international terrorism, the pervasive influence of the one remaining super-power (i.e. the USA), and the fomenting of a 'New World Order' (Kagan, 2003) are yet to be fully recognized. Nor has the connection between mental health policy and human rights been given sufficient attention.

Concerns about human protection, respect, dignity, tolerance, and betterment have a history that stretches beyond ancient Greece and Rome to the very beginnings of social gatherings. No societal epoch, whether hunter-gatherer, agricultural, industrial, or post-modern, can endure without some degree of either expressed or intuitive regard for the continued existence, well-being, and advancement of its populace.

However, rarely has such concern applied throughout a society or been viewed as pertinent to external societies. Indeed, it was not until the mid-20th century, with the formation of the United Nations (UN), and the Universal Declaration of Human Rights, that such humanitarian matters became formalized principles with universal application:

- All human beings are born free and equal in dignity and rights. They are endowed with reason and conscience and should act towards one another in a spirit of brotherhood. (Article 1)

- Everyone is entitled to all the rights and freedoms set forth in this declaration, without distinction of any kind, such as race, colour, sex, language, religion, political or other opinion, national or social origin, property, birth or other status. (Extract, Article 2)

- Everyone has the right to life, liberty and security of person. (Article 3)
                                                              (United Nations, 1948)

Agreement to these basic human rights has been virtually universal. That is the point of United Nations membership – to formulate and sanction transnational social programmes that lead to a better, more peaceful world. However, far from improvements in the quality of people's lives, and how they are dealt with by those in power, there is a:

... growing disparity between the almost globally accepted standard for the protection of human rights and the daily denial of those basic rights to millions of people.
                                                        (Dunne and Wheeler, 1999: ix)

All too often people have no voice in the political process, suffer discrimination and are tortured or even killed by their own governments. They face bloodshed, rape, genocide, and ethnic cleansing; they live in desperate deprivation alongside ostentatious opulence, suffer disease, malnutrition and low life expectancy, while the privileged of their country or populations, merely a few hours' airplane journey away, increase their material wealth and life-span dramatically. The level of inequality worldwide has been described by the UN as 'grotesque', and inequality is growing, not narrowing (United Nations, 2002). At least three billion people live in abject poverty, and poverty is a serious barrier to mental health (WHO, 1999). Poor people get poor justice; poor mentally disordered people may get the poorest justice.

Following the bombing of the New York World Trade Center on September 11, 2001, mature liberal-democratic states such as the USA, Australia, and Britain have introduced 'post-liberal' legislation, for example, detainment without trial. Hyper-social control of this nature may be necessary to prevent other atrocities in Western countries, but undermines the cultural practices, including human rights, it is being implemented to preserve. Post-liberal laws also apply to other types of 'risky' people. For instance, in the UK pre-emptive detainment has been advocated for individuals diagnosed with certain 'dangerous' mental conditions. Moreover, there is no guarantee that liberal-democratic governments will not either dilute or revoke existing human rights legislation.

As part of the debate surrounding human rights and human development it has been asserted that the best way of promoting human development and safeguarding human freedom and dignity is to build strong and deep forms of democratic governance at all levels of society (United Nations, 2002: 1). It is argued that the promotion of human development, including human rights, is only possible when governance systems are democratically accountable, enabling people to participate in the debates and decisions that shape their lives. However, we would add an important qualification here. While democratic governance may be a precondition for political and civil freedoms and the right to participate, it is no guarantee. As the UN's Human Development Report 2002 acknowledges:

> The links between democracy and human development are not automatic: when a small elite dominates economic and political decisions, the link between democracy and equity can be broken.
>
> (United Nations, 2002: 3)

The UN's Declaration of Human Rights (1948) makes reference to the universal human right of access to adequate health care. However, the World Health Organization records that, of a sampled 185 developed and developing countries, for 70% of people there is only one psychiatrist and for 44% one psychiatric nurse per 100,000 of the population. Less than 1% of the health budget for the majority of the countries in the sample is designated for mental health; there are no community care resources for 37%; and 40% did not have a mental health policy at all. That is, in the 21st century, and accepting the belated (in terms of the history of human civilization) acknowledgement of human rights, a large minority of people in the world will not receive any help or defective assistance if they become mentally unhealthy.

Principles for the protection and treatment of people suffering from mental disorder have been proclaimed by the General Assembly of the UN. These are morally laudable, socially pervasive, and penetrating. For example, people with mental disorder are expected to have access to the best available medical care determined by their needs, be diagnosed without any political interference and shielded from exploitation, discrimination and stigma (United Nations, 1991).

However, not only was it as late as the 1990s that the principles were adopted, but also the UN still accepts that there are circumstances when involuntary incarceration and enforced treatment (possibly psychosurgical), restraint, and seclusion can be used. Moreover, without momentous political change internationally involving ideological and budgetary commitment to commensurate health and social care – these ideals remain largely unrealizable.

The WHO has affirmed that the human rights of people with mental disorders continue, in the 21st century, to be violated in psychiatric institutions, where they may reside in grim and unhygienic conditions, exposed to harmful methods of 'care'. Outside of institutions, the attitudes of the community and the press persist in being damaging to the self-esteem of the users of mental health services, undermining the possibility of their social inclusion with respect to employment, housing and education.

Paradoxically, much of what is advocated by the UN and WHO rests on specific, and therefore skewed, concepts and constructions of human rights and health. That is, there is an inherent promulgation of principles and policies that are consanguine with North American and European social procedures, philosophies, laws, and the discourse of scientific medicine. There is also categorical support from the UN and WHO (and other trans-national agencies such as the Council of Europe, 2000) for the implementation of mental health legislation. This is justified on the basis that laws are open to scrutiny and can be used to protect mentally disordered people by enshrining human rights tenets. For example, a recent WHO mental health and human rights project states:

> Legislation enables the codification and consolidation of the fundamental principles, values, aims and objectives of mental health policies and programmes. It provides a legal framework to ensure that critical issues affecting the lives of people with mental disorders, both in mental health facilities and in the broader community context, are addressed.
>
> (WHO, 2003: 1)

Conversely, laws can just as easily be utilized for the apparent safekeeping of the community, the beneficiaries of social inequity, and the furtherance of medical hegemony, to the detriment of individual freedom and alternative approaches to mental health. For example, referring to mentally disordered criminal offenders, the UN General Assembly resolutions that list principles aimed at improving mental health care states:

> All such persons should receive the best available mental health care ... Domestic law may authorize a court or other competent authority, acting on the basis of competent and independent medical advice, to order that such persons to be admitted to a mental health facility.
>
> (Principle 20, United Nations, 1991)

But secure mental health facilities may not have the capacity to offer the most appropriate treatment, particularly if this is 'social' rather than medical. Large numbers of mentally disordered offenders are incarcerated in prisons rather than facilities specializing in the complex needs of such people. In prison, mental health care, if available at all, will be very limited. Furthermore, an acceptance of the supremacy of local law presupposes that such laws venerate human rights. Local law in the most human rights conscious country in the world (the USA) allows for execution by hanging, lethal injection, or electric chair of sane and mentally disordered citizens. Perversely, and reminiscent of Joseph Heller's *Catch-22*, successful medical intervention may have the unintended consequence of condemning a mentally disordered person to State-sponsored (lawful) killing:

> A US appeal court has ruled that a mentally ill man who has been on death row for 25 years is sane enough when on medication to be executed. Charles Singleton would be too insane to qualify for execution without drugs.
>
> (Associated Press, 2003)

Human rights abuse of mentally disordered people, particularly those who are without the social capital to challenge mistreatment as a consequence of the severity of their illness, and who may be residing (voluntarily or involuntarily) in unregulated establishments, can be manifestly brutal. Examples can be given from across the globe, and some are referred to in this book. Others include the results of an investigation by Mental Disability International into mental health care in Kosovo, which reported incidents of rape, violence, and the disgusting sleeping arrangements for residents (Jennings, 2002). Bulgaria, at the heart of Europe and an applicant for European Union membership, has also come under fierce opprobrium by Amnesty International for disrespect of rudimentary principles of care in psychiatric hospitals, and cruel and degrading treatment. Amnesty International has alleged that patients were malnourished, living in freezing temperatures, caged, beaten, and subjected to 'unmodified' electroconvulsive therapy, that is, without anaesthetic (Amnesty International, 2002).

There are also many cases of the violation of psychiatry, for example, in China under Jiang Zemin (now retired as Communist Party Chairman but remaining as Commander in Chief of the military) and in the former Union of Soviet Socialist Republics. Despotic regimes and movements of both communist and fascist hue use psychiatry as a tool of social oppression today and in the past:

> For dictator General Francisco Franco's chief psychiatrist, Dr. Antonio Vallejo Nagera, it must have seemed obvious. If the generalissimo and his fellow right-wing rebels in the Spanish civil war were crusaders for justice, God and the truth, then their left-wing opponents had to be mad, psychotic or at least congenitally subnormal ... Little surprise then, that he classified almost a third of the English [International Brigade] prisoners as 'mental retards'.

Another third were deemed to be suffering degenerative mental illnesses that were turning them into schizoids, paranoids or psychopaths. Their fall into Marxism [argued Nagera] was, in turn, exacerbated by the fact that 29% were also considered 'social imbeciles'.

(Tremlett, 2002)

Cuba has been accused of using psychiatry to re-classify political opponents of Fidel Castro. It is alleged that since the 1960s some 'political recidivists', who did not succumb to 're-education', were diagnosed as mentally disordered by psychiatrists working with the security service (Brown and Lago, 1991; Lago, 2000). Cases have been cited of 'psychiatric torture' such as the excessive and inappropriate use of psychotic medication and ECT (Stride, 1997). Ironically, this country has a well-deserved international reputation for investment in health (and educational) services in defiance of an extremely low gross national product.

Our interest, and the rationale for the book, is to reflect on the 'global' intentions of the UN/WHO and ask what approaches to mental health policy are evident in a selection of countries, and what are the concomitant human rights issues. A series of case studies from across the world is presented by experts on the relevant country. Many of the authors are or have been involved in determining mental health policy at the supra-national level within such organizations as the UN and the WHO.

In most cases the countries have been chosen on the basis of their geographical location (i.e. to ensure that there is a spread of exemplars from both the developed and developing world). In other instances selection has been based on an influential historical role (i.e. the British Empire 'exported' its incarceration techniques to many parts of the world during the 19th century), a unique approach to managing the mentally disordered (i.e. Italy's programme of de-institutionalization), or because of special (and horrific) circumstances that have serious and long-lasting implications for mental health and human rights (i.e. war-torn Mozambique).

We also purposefully sought diversity in political regime and human development. Chapters 1 to 4 report on developments in highly industrialized liberal democratic states – the UK, USA, Australia and Italy – where governments have invested heavily in overhauling mental health policies and services. All four of these countries are listed in the High Human Development band of the Human Development Index (HDI; United Nations, 2002).

Chapters 5 and 6 cover Egypt and India respectively, two developing countries in which mental health reform is taking place against a backdrop of relative political stability. Chapter 7 on Brazil outlines developments in mental policy and practice in a country making the transition from military dictatorship to liberal democracy. All three of these countries are listed in the Medium Human Development band of the HDI.

Table 1 Selected Countries' Human Development Index (HDI) Rank and Score[1]

Country	HDI Score	HDI Rank
Australia	0.939	5
USA	0.939	6
UK	0.928	13
Italy	0.913	20
Russia	0.781	60
Brazil	0.757	73
China	0.726	96
Egypt	0.642	115
India	0.577	124
Mozambique	0.322	170

[1] The Human Development Index (HDI) is a measure of development devised by analysts working in the United Nations Development Program (UNDP). A country's HDI is calculated with reference to three indices: life expectancy, education and income. The HDI value is expressed as a figure somewhere between 0 and 1.

Chapters 8 and 9, reporting on Russia and China respectively, address issues surrounding the use of psychiatry as an instrument for achieving the political ends of the state. In Russia, democratization following the end of the Soviet empire coincided with moves to separate psychiatry from state control. However, the pace of reform slowed markedly with the differing political situation ushered in by the war in Chechnya. The Chinese case study outlines the means by which psychiatry may be drawn into the state-sponsored persecution of what are seen as 'troublesome' groups, in this case the practitioners of Falun Gong. Both Russia and China are listed in the Medium Human Development band of the HDI.

Chapter 10 on Mozambique outlines the challenges faced in establishing mental health care in a country emerging from a period of political instability and internal armed conflict. One of the World's poorest nations, Mozambique is ranked toward the bottom of the Low Human Development band of the HDI.

The Human Development Index scores and ranks of the countries included in the book are presented in Table 1.

It is also true that in part the choice of which countries to include was decreed by serendipity. We are very lucky to get the expertise contained within this book and we are grateful to all of the contributors.

A format for the shaping of the chapters was suggested by us as editors (i.e. coverage of the historical background of mental health policy, the contemporary situation, and if possible examples of individuals' experiences of the mental health system). However, the authors have embraced a variety of styles. While many draw out explicitly themes and abuses (for example, China's labelling of Falun Gong members as 'mad'), others have indicated implicitly what are or have been the contexts and consequences for human rights (for example, market-orientated health care in the USA). These stylistic deviations may simply be the result of 'academic independence', i.e. authors deciding to follow a plan that they believe is more effective in delivering what messages they consider important. It may also imply that the assumption of an internationally shared discourse of mental health/illness and human rights is not, and can never be, ratified.

References

Amnesty International (2002) Grave Lack of Respect for Basic Human Rights of People with Mental Disabilities in Bulgaria. News Service 175, EUR 15/013/2002. London: Amnesty International.

Associated Press (2003) Killer can be Executed Because Drugs Make Him Sane. http://www.ananova.com/news/story/sm_749575.html?menu=3Dnews.latesheadli=

Brown CJ, Lago AM (1991) The Politics of Psychiatry in Revolutionary Cuba. New Brunswick, NJ: Transaction.

Council of Europe (2000) White Paper on Mental Health and Human Rights. http://www.doh.gov.uk/mha/coe.htm

Dunne T, Wheeler N (Eds.) (1999) Human Rights and Global Politics. Cambridge: Cambridge University Press.

Jennings C (2002) Kosovo Mental Care Abuses Revealed. The Daily Telegraph, 9 August.

Kagan K (2001) Paradise and Power: America and Europe in the New World Order. London: Atlantic Books.

Lago AM (2000) Loss of Life Resulting from the Cuban Revolution: On Cuban Psychiatric Abuse. http://www.geocities.com/policraticus/on_cuban_psychiatric_abuse.html

Stride JT (1997) Task Force Seeks Update on Misuse of Psychiatry in Cuba. CubaNet – News. http://64.21.33.164/Cnews/y97/jan97/25mazor.html

Tremlett C (2002) Marxists are Retards. The Guardian, 1 November.

United Nations (1948) Universal Declaration of Human Rights. New York: United Nations.

United Nations (1991) Principles for the Protection of Persons with Mental Illness and the Improvement of Mental Health Care. New York: United Nations High Commissioner for Human Rights.

United Nations (2002) Human Development Report 2002. New York: United Nations Development Programme.

World Health Organization (1999) Raising Awareness, Fighting Stigma, Improving Care. Press release WHO/67, 12 November. Geneva: WHO.

World Health Organization (2001) Mapping Mental Health Resources Around the World. Geneva: WHO.

World Health Organization (2003) WHO Mental Health and Human Rights Project. Geneva: WHO.

CHAPTER ONE

UK mental health policy: Chaos and control

PETER MORRALL

Introduction

United Kingdom (UK) mental health policy in the 21st century is characterized by chaos and control.

Much of the chaos has been inherited from a policy deluge towards the end of the last century. Today mental health practitioners in the UK are attempting to cope with a plethora of guidelines, programmes, procedures, legislation, and pressure group demands that is inherently contradictory, politically expedient, asymmetric, and pragmatically unrealizable. But no matter how shambolic, mental health policy has now a distinct core property: the increased regulation of mad behaviour.

To begin with, the UK is not 'united' in terms of health programmes or the law. Scotland has its own parliament, and Wales has its legislative assembly. Moreover, there remains a myriad of tensions and disputes involving the various mental health professional groups over hierarchical positions and legitimate working areas.

Evidence-based practice co-exists with evidence of practice flaws, scientific rigour with a continued allegiance to 'intuition' and 'experience'. Human rights legislation has further muddied the waters in the rising and turbulent sea of policies. There is an indefinite period of uncertainty concerning the day-to-day legal management of mentally disordered people within the health system as 'case law' unfolds. The old mental health laws had been discredited for many years and are in need of reform (Eastman, 1996; Royal College of Psychiatrists, 2000), but reform of these laws has been highly controversial (Laurance, 2002; Morris, 2002).

Large numbers of people with mental health disorders have also become ensnared in the criminal justice system. A considerable proportion of the prison population has been recognized as suffering from mental disorder (either as a condition existing prior to conviction or caused by imprisonment), but do not receive adequate or (in many cases) any treatment.

Incredibly, there is an ongoing debate over what basic skills and training mental health nurses, the largest occupational discipline involved in mental health care, should have at their disposal. After nearly two centuries of 'keepers', 'attendants', and 'nurses' caring for mentally disordered people we have to re-affirm what is a 'capable practitioner' (Sainsbury Centre, 2000a), presumably because 'incapability' is pervasive.

Juxtaposed with chaos, existing and projected ordinances on mental health practice reproduce the post-liberal division of 'self-regulated individualism' and 'demonization' found in society at large. State-orchestrated control measures sub-divide the participating citizen, with social rights and responsibilities, from the social deviant, stripped of his/her rights due to irresponsible conduct. The psychiatric disciplines divide the mentally disordered population into those that can be encouraged to self-regulate (through the talking therapies, and mood-mediating medication) and those who are perceived to be ineligible for self-regulation (the severely psychotic, and the psychopath).

While other types of health care users are not immune from the side-effects of policy obfuscation (for example, cancer, coronary, and accident and emergency services have all been recognized as feckless), the customers of the mad industry are especially vulnerable. They are, despite empowerment and advocacy movements (which, ironically, can contribute to the muddle), unable in the main, due to the very properties of their disorder, to contend with, or find suitable alternatives to, such state-sponsored inefficiency. The state (in the form of government departments – in particular the Department of Health and the Home Office – and agencies of social control – especially psychiatric medicine and nursing) could be considered to be propagating large-scale abuse. Not caring for the 'unreasonable' reasonably (i.e. by not having coherent service provision, and at the same time focusing on 'control') is to negate the human rights of mentally disordered people as a collectivity.

Historical background

The designation of insanity, until quite recently in the history of Western civilization, was based on the notion that the mad were irredeemably distinguishable from the rest of humanity. They were a separate *genus* from that of 'normal' people, essentially 'wild beasts', and as such were either to be excluded from the jurisdiction of the courts, given access to whatever mental health provision was present, or dealt with by separate laws and forms of discipline (Robinson, 1996).

But while the dichotomy between 'humans' and 'beasts' had sprung from ancient Greece, during the Middle Ages in Europe the intolerance and bigotry of the Christian church, and the superstitious absurdities and cruelties of feudal life, were to produce a conflation of categories of behaviour. What we may now consider to be behaviour that was a challenge to the church or nobility, or was at root madness, had the potential to be reconfigured as sorcery, and as such could have terrible consequences for the accused – torture, damnation, and execution (Gibson, 1999).

Busfield (1996) suggests that there have been three phases in the evolution of formal mental health policy in England. Prior to the 17th century, in the main the mad, if confined (that is, if not cared for by their families), were sent to bridewells (Tudor 'houses of correction'), common gaols, and workhouses. Much of the cause for incarceration, argues Busfield, can be traced to the Poor Laws, which reduced the possibility of financial support in the community and non-institutional facilities.

The building of workhouses began in the 1630s. The Poor Law Act of 1601 dictated that each parish must take responsibility for its elderly, sick, idiots, and lunatics. The Act of Settlement 1662 restricted what was already very limited support for only those who were *bona fide* residents. Most market towns in England built a workhouse as the solution to the problem of looking after its social outcasts (Sheppard, 2000).

Until the 17th century, Bethlem in London was the only specialized institution for the mad throughout Europe (Andrews et al., 1997). Bethlem was founded in 1247 as a priory to the Order of St Mary of Bethlehem. Originally operating as a 'hospice', it accepted lunatics from 1377 onwards. However, there were only 44 patients in Bethlem by 1642, although in 1676 a re-sited Bethlem could take up to 150 patients, who had to be poor and assessed as curable (Sheppard, 2000).

The 17th century (Busfield's first phase) saw the separation of healing for the wealthy-mad from the impoverished-mad with the establishment of commercially run madhouses (Busfield, 1996). The segregation of the mad who were poor from the rest of society was promoted further in the 18th century with the creation of the charitable voluntary asylums.

Busfield's second phase was the building of large numbers of public asylums in the 19th century, which had the effect of normalizing the separation of madness from both normality and other forms of social deviance. Following the 1845 Lunacy Act in England, local authorities were forced to provide for the mad through a massive public building programme. Asylums were to house more than 100,000 inmates by 1900. Moreover, the public asylums were given wide powers to compulsorily detain the mad, which engendered their custodial character (Busfield, 1996).

Asylums offered the medical specialist the opportunity to deliver and experiment with new treatments on a captive audience (Porter, 2002). Psychiatric treatments in the 19th century involved stimulants, sedatives, emetics, purgatives, bloodletting, cold and hot baths (without the religious overtones), mechanical restraints, and electric shocks. However, 'moral treatment', supported by lay benefactors and religious groups such as the Quakers, was to compete with organic medicine. The Retreat in York was founded in 1796 by William Tuke, one of many philanthropic tea merchants of the time and member of the Society of Friends. This private asylum was built and organized counter to those run by medical practitioners (such as the York Asylum, some three miles away). Moral management held that the mad could be brought back to reason if handled more humanely but nevertheless 'trained' to be normal (Porter, 1987).

Employing a technique that has served the profession of medicine extremely well, rather than deriding this popular approach, doctors encompassed moral therapy within their assortment of procedures. The effect of 'medicalizing' moral treatment was to leave psychiatrists '...firmly in charge of the whole enterprise' (Johnstone, 2000: 149). From the point of view of the psychiatrists, this move gave their patients the benefit of both scientific treatment and compassionate care.

The Victorian asylums, and those that came after in the 20th century, were an enormous financial investment for governments of the day, one which could not be replicated today. They were built on the back of high ideals. The mad could partake of fresh air in rural surroundings, in the extensive grounds and gardens that most of the asylums had procured (Gittins, 1998). Food and water were comparatively fresh, clean, and nutritious. Recreation and rest were encouraged, as was (with the introduction of 'moral therapy') industrious activity when the inmate was perceived to be in need of such to aid her/his recovery.

It was not until the 1930s, the third phase in Busfield's historical taxonomy, that effective reform took place, allowing for voluntary admission, when welfare support increased significantly the chances of non-institutional care, and hence increasingly the likelihood of discharge. Competing ideas of madness waxed and waned depending on the context in which services were provided. Asylums offered the medical profession the opportunity to reinforce the status and use of physical methods of treatment.

A new age of community care arrived in the early part of the 20th century in Europe and the USA with the Mental Hygiene Movement (Goodwin, 1997). In Britain outpatient clinics were established, and further medical treatments (for example, insulin therapy and electro-convulsant therapy) developed. A major achievement for psychiatry in France and the USA was the discovery of drugs in the 1950s that could dampen down psychotic symptoms. The discovery of these drugs, while not solely the cause of the demise of institutional care (Miller and Rose, 1986), enabled previously deranged patients to at least spend large amounts of time 'on leave' or possibly to be discharged.

Medical diagnostic technology developed rapidly during the 1980s, for example, computerized axial tomography, magnetic resonance imaging, neuroimaging, photomicrography, positron emission tomography, and single photon emission tomography. Moreover, a new wave of drugs such as the selective serotonin re-uptake inhibitors (SSRIs) and 'atypical' anti-psychotics have entered the psychiatrist's arsenal of physical methods. However, not only had psychology already had a major impact, emanating from the work of Sigmund Freud (1856–1939), but also social approaches became possible (Busfield, 1996).

The contemporary situation

In the UK, community care became most explicit as the overriding mental health policy during the 1960s (Johnstone, 2000). A sharp reduction in hospital beds from the peak of 155,000 during the 1950s in Britain continued throughout the 1960s and 1970s. The number of in-patient beds was only 36,000 by the end of the 20th century (McCulloch et al., 2000). The emphasis for treatment moved from institutional psychiatric services to primary care (largely delivered by general practitioners and community mental health teams).

However, community services were never able to compensate for the loss of many of the large institutions. Government finances previously spent on running the large institutions were not effectively transferred to local authorities to fund community care facilities. If local authorities took it upon themselves to build up such facilities they were penalized financially by the government (Beardshaw and Morgan, 1990).

As a consequence, the remaining in-patient services came under intense pressure. For example, admissions have risen from 200,000 in 1983 to 270,100 in 1995 (Sainsbury Centre, 1998). The number of compulsory admissions of patients (under the 1983 Mental Health Act) to National Health Service (NHS) hospitals rose from 15,400 in 1987–1988 to 25,100 in 1997–1998 (Department of Health, 1998a). During March of 1998, 12,700 patients were detained in hospital, of whom 1,300 were in high security psychiatric (special) hospitals.

The financial burden of mental disorder in the UK is greater than that of the defence budget even in times of war (such as the 2003 conflict with Iraq), and represents 4% of the gross domestic product. The calculation of £32 billion (for the year 1996–1997), by health economists at the Institute of Psychiatry in London, is based on adding together the figures for: wasted productivity (including that lost through suicide); social security payments health, local authority, and criminal justice services; and informal care (Brindle, 1997).

No matter what the financial burden, however, there has been general agreement about the poor state of mental health services. The clinical psychologist and critic of the psychiatric profession Lucy Johnstone (2000) has argued that psychiatry is in a condition of 'transition'. Senior 'establishment' figures such as Graham Thornicroft (1998), Professor of Community Psychiatry at the Institute of Psychiatry, have described the policies for the mentally disordered as 'half-minded'. The press have characterized the mental health service as in 'turmoil' (Fletcher, 1995) and a 'system under strain' which is 'stumbling into the "lock-'em-up and drug-'em-up" policies of a shameful past' (Laurance, 2003).

Overload

The mayhem in mental health policy is signified through a never-ending deluge of initiatives, decrees, and recommendations. In the last few decades in Britain, the mental health aspect of the NHS has had to introduce:

- a 'management-led' rather than 'profession-led' hierarchy;
- an internal market in health care provision whereby, for example, purchasers (commissioners) and providers of health care services are separated, and general practitioners as 'fund-holders' can procure alternative clinical services;
- a distinction between 'social' and 'health' care;
- community mental health teams;
- methods of engaging with the severely mentally disordered people who have multiple and long-term health and social requirements;
- the care programme approach, case management, and key workers;
- supervision registers;
- non-custodial care and treatment to mentally disordered offenders;
- plans to reduce morbidity and suicide rates among the mentally ill;
- amendments to the Mental Health Act 1983;
- tools for assessing and managing the risk of violence;
- inter-agency partnerships;
- processes and guidelines to empower users and carers;
- the auditing of clinical practice;
- recommendations from a succession of reviews concerning the education, roles, and competencies and capabilities of nurses;
- sensitive measures for ethnic and faith diversity;
- various types of 'crises' and 'preventative' teams;
- primary care mental health graduate workers, and general practitioners and nurses with 'special interests' in primary mental health care;
- 24-hour services; and
- evidence-based practice.

Moreover, in the late 1990s a long-term updating of the NHS began, designed to improve buildings and equipment, invest in staff training, and procure and develop leading-edge information technology. Added to this major overhaul of the whole state-run health care system and the subsequent drive for 'cultural change' in the NHS through the instigation of 'Foundation Hospitals' intended to boost patient choice (Milburn, 2003), the Department of Health launched its objective to renovate all mental health provision including legislation.

Opprobrium

Confirming prolonged public anxiety about the competence of such groups as social workers, general practitioners, psychiatrists, and psychiatric nurses, the mental health disciplines have been criticized severely for not 'pulling together' (Sainsbury Centre, 1997). This level of concern has also been expressed about in-patient services. In a study of 118 psychiatric units in England and Wales (representing 47% of the total number of in-patient services in NHS trusts), two major failings were revealed (Ford et al., 1998). First, there was considerable pressure on the acute services (in terms of being able to admit more patients than there are beds), but in part this was created by poor management strategies. Specifically, the study concluded that the policy of sending patients who are compulsorily detained under the Mental Health Act of 1983 on short or unspecified leave into the community resulted in these beds being unusable for other patients requiring admission as it was unknown when the 'detained' patients would return. Second, not only was there a serious difficulty in staffing the psychiatric units, which resulted in the over-use of 'bank' or 'agency' nurses, but also there was little interaction with patients in a sizeable minority of the institutions visited.

In another survey of care in acute psychiatric wards, information was gathered from over 200 patients about their experiences (Sainsbury Centre, 1998). The conclusions of the investigative team were that although the immediate mental state of the patients improved during their stay in hospital, as measured by the patients' own accounts and objective assessment (using the Brief Psychiatric Rating Scale), they had not had their long-term and individual needs met. The study concluded that 'hospital care was a non-therapeutic intervention' as most of the patients became bored due to the absence of structured activity, had little privacy, and many feared for their personal safety. A recommendation of the study was that acute hospital services should be completely reconstructed.

In research that repeated studies of acute mental health services conducted in the 1980s, Higgins et al. (1999) interviewed over 100 staff and 52 patients, and observed ward activity in 11 sites. These researchers concluded that the education psychiatric nurses receive does not equip them adequately for working in acute settings. For example, concern was expressed by those interviewed that newly qualified nurses did not have relevant and practical skills for the clinical situations they had to deal with. Higgins et al. also recorded that the increase in time that senior ward staff spent on paperwork and office duties was 'astonishing'. The most senior of these nurses in 1985 spent one-third of their time on this type of work. By 1996, nearly three-quarters of their time was occupied with administrative tasks. Axiomatically, these nurses were in direct contact with patients in 1996 for less than 6% of their working day, compared with nearly 30% in 1986. As a consequence:

> ... many [patients] had only a passing relationship with nurses who were typ-ically in the office writing, telephoning or dealing with unexpected incidents in the ward. This resulted in the boredom reported by many patients who, when in hospital, felt that they were often left to their own devices.
>
> (Higgins et al., 1999: 154)

A report by the Standing Nursing and Midwifery Advisory Committee (SNMAC, 1999), a statutory body, concluded that there was a deficit in nurs-ing leadership and skills among staff working in acute in-patient care, and that these areas were becoming increasingly custodial rather than thera-peutic in orientation. The authors of the report suggest that care is not planned in a co-ordinated manner either among the professions or across the settings such as hospital and community, and users and carers are not involved in care processes. Moreover, nurses are not basing their practice on 'evidence'. The latter conclusion of the SNMAC is echoed by the Sainsbury Centre, but this is not a problem confined to the mental health arena:

> In common with much health care, only a small proportion of mental health care is currently based on the available evidence.
>
> (Sainsbury Centre, 2001a: 3)

McCulloch et al. (2000) observe that the mental health system has changed from one entirely of in-patient care to one of an in-patient service that deals only with the most 'acutely' disturbed and needy people. Not only does this mean that acute services are, according to the former president of the Royal College of Psychiatrists, 'inadequate' and environ-mentally 'awful' (quoted in BBC News, 2001), but also that community services are not fully staffed with the appropriate range of mental health practitioners and yet are carrying huge caseloads. They are, therefore, unable to provide what may be indicated as necessary in the patients' care plan. Users of the mental health system become enmeshed in the 'revolv-ing door' of admission and re-admission, with only medication, simplistic interpersonal therapy, and containment offered to satisfy complex needs.

Such a state of affairs has had the side-effect of violence becoming endemic in the mental health system. Many members of staff experience daily violent outbursts by patients in acute wards and forensic facilities. Violence, either in the form of verbal aggression or physical assault, is directed towards other patients, but mainly towards members of staff (two out of every three incidents). However, despite such regularity, few nurses have undergone comprehensive training in the management of violence (SNMAC, 1999; UKCC, 2002).

This poor condition of the mental health system in the UK has resulted in immense dissatisfaction among users and carers (McCulloch et al., 2000). There is also a pressing concern over the recruitment and retention of mental health nurses and psychiatrists (Royal College of Psychiatrists, 2000; Sainsbury Centre, 2000b).

Restoration

Improving the mental health services was proclaimed a priority by the Labour Government, and a three-stage strategy put forward (Department of Health, 2001a). This strategy incorporated a number of already published (although not always implemented) policies.

First, more money is to be spent on mental health services to provide more secure beds (up to 500), extra 24-hour beds (over 300), and 170 assertive outreach teams. Moreover, under the NHS Plan (Department of Health, 2000) – yet another reorganization of provision – a further £300 million will be invested in mental health services for the years 2001–2004, with extra monies for ward refurbishment, dual diagnoses provision (i.e. drug/alcohol and severe mental illness), and child and adolescent services.

Second, the inequalities that exist in health provision are to be addressed (the so-called 'post-code lottery'). Following recommendation in the document *Modernising Mental Health Services* (Department of Health, 1998b), the Mental Health National Service Framework (NSF) sets out standards of care for the whole of the country (Department of Health, 1999). The NHS Plan contains other initiatives that attempt to close any remaining gaps in services. A new government co-ordinating agency, the National Institute for Mental Health Services in England (NIMHSE) is to be established. The purpose of NIMHSE is to improve the quality, organization, and range of facilities available to mental health service users, and is to be headed up by a mental health policy 'Tsar', Professor Louis Appleby, National Director for Mental Health (Department of Health, 2001b). NIMHSE will also focus on accruing and disseminating research evidence to support effective treatment and care. Appleby has also been appointed as chair to the Mental Health Task Force (MHTF), set up by the government to ensure that the objectives of the National Service Framework for Mental Health and the National Plan are met (Department of Health, 2002a).

Third, is the new legal framework for mental health meant to replace the Mental Health Act 1983 (Department of Health, 2002d)? There is recognition that the vast majority of people who use the mental health service in the UK do so voluntarily. However, for those with any mental disorder that is either permanent or temporary and which disturbs mental functioning, and who are either unable or unwilling to seek care and treatment, then legislation has to be available to prevent their condition worsening, or to prevent them from harming themselves or other people. Such legislation, above and beyond common law, therefore includes powers to restrict personal liberty, alongside a commitment to inform patients about what these powers entail, free legal representation, and access to review processes and independent advocacy services.

Incoherence

A major problem, however, with this strategy is incoherence. The policies it incorporates were not designed originally to be part of the strategy and therefore do not necessarily 'fit' the tenets or application of that programme. There is overlap of purpose, and financial accountability and distribution of funding. Different agencies and disciplines (for example, state and voluntary; health and social services) with perhaps competing agendas, and at alternative levels (i.e. local and central government), are responsible for executing the strategy. The supply of mental health care is not well integrated, and mentally disordered people frequently find that their needs are not met due to bureaucratic obstacles undermining effective co-ordination between the multiple agencies (McCulloch et al., 2000). Specific areas within any particular policy may have labyrinthine systems of sub-agencies advising and taking responsibility for their operation. For example, six 'action teams' were appointed to deliver the NHS Plan. The MHTF has created the Mental Health Promotion Project (MHPP) to champion NSF Standard 1 (of seven standards overall), which refers to health promotion, as well as challenging discrimination against, and encouraging the social inclusion of, mentally disordered people (Department of Health, 2001c). Preventing suicide is another major part of the brief of the MHPP. However, suicide prevention is tackled not only as Standard 7 of the NSF, but specifically within the National Confidential Inquiry into Suicide and Homicide (Appleby, 2001), the NHS Plan, the Acute In-patient Care Strategy (Department of Health, 2002b), and the National Suicide Prevention Strategy (Department of Health, 2002c). Moreover, the National Institute for Clinical Practice, the Royal College of Psychiatrists, the prison service, and the NIMHSE have produced, or intend to produce, their own guidelines on suicide prevention/risk assessment.

The objective of the MHPP to promote the mental well-being of the whole of the population is laudable but impracticable. Social change on a massive scale and a concomitant budget would have to be sought to deal with the psychological ill-effects of poverty, unemployment, overwork, divorce, a failing transport infrastructure, terrorism, crime, racism, sexism, ageism, and the idiosyncratic stress factors that affect each individual.

Variations in care (the post-code lottery) are not only being tackled by the NSF, MHTF, NHS Plan, and NIMHSE, but also through the quality control system of 'clinical governance' organized by yet another government agency, the Commission for Health Improvement (CHI). CHI is responsible for clinical governance reviews in every part of the NHS (England and Wales), including mental health, to ensure that the highest level of care is delivered (Commission for Health Improvement, 2002). However, another agency, the National Institute for Clinical Excellence (NICE), directs policy on, for example, drug treatment, concentrating on cost-effectiveness and efficacy.

Controversy over the major policy changes abounds. For example, the prestigious Institute of Psychiatry in London, in one of a series of public debates about contemporary mental health care policy, raised the issue of whether or not the NHS Plan, the cornerstone of government policy, was a genuine attempt to improve provision. The title of the debate was 'Plan or Sham? This house believes that the NHS Plan will transform psychiatric care in England for the better' (Institute of Psychiatry, 2001). The debate concerned whether or not this seemingly fundamental and radical alteration in how mental health services are organized and delivered was the result not of priorities in care but politics and therefore full of 'gimmicks' and financially unsustainable. In particular, the NHS Plan contains proposals for a significant expansion in forensic psychiatric facilities for people with 'dangerous severe personality disorder' (DSPD), a new category of mental disorder, as well as crisis teams, assertive outreach teams, and early onset of psychosis teams. Professor Appleby supported the motion. It was contested by Professor Sir David Goldberg, formerly of the Institute of Psychiatry, and presently Chief Executive of the National Schizophrenia Fellowship. Scepticism won the day, with the non-representative audience of mental health professionals, service users, and carers voting (narrowly) against the motion (MacCabe, 2001).

There is also a volatile wider policy context that directly affects the way in which mental health services can function. For example, the creation of primary health care trusts (PHCTs) impinges on the specialism of mental health, traditionally a service mainly concerned with secondary and tertiary care. Many PHCTs are attempting to incorporate within their organizational structures elements of mental health provision (for example, in-patient facilities) that previously would not be considered to be in the primary care domain. There is concern that PHCTs have little understanding of the mental health agenda, with few of those aspiring to administer such services having the necessary expertise, and being unable to offer sufficient care for people with severe mental disorders (Sainsbury Centre, 2001b).

There is the further complication of private psychiatric care, such as the 20 clinics operated by Priory Healthcare. Private care is not an insignificant proportion of the total mental health service provision, half of which is used by the NHS to compensate for its own inability to provide sufficient in-patient care (McCullock et al., 2000).

Furthermore, mental disorder is inherently a hotly contested arena (Coppock and Hopton, 2000). Contemporary mental health is replete with rival treatments: old and new anti-psychotic and anti-depressant drugs; 'talking therapies' (for example, psychoanalysis, cognitive–behavioural therapy, neuro-linguistic programming, brief therapy, humanistic counselling); psychosurgery; electroconvulsant therapy. There is also much disputation over what counts as good practice, despite the prevalence of the evidence-based practice doctrine, with the randomized control trial featuring as the 'gold standard' of valid and reliable research. NICE has produced 'good practice' guidance for schizophrenia that aims to accommodate alternative treatment modes, agencies, and levels (National Institute for Clinical Excellence, 2002). However, this is comprehensive, complex, and, as it is only guidance, may be ignored by practitioners, particularly if the suggested 'pathway' does not embrace their epistemological leanings, skills, and resources.

Moreover, the dominant profession, psychiatry, is not unified over how to deliver mental health care. Anti-psychiatry, a movement that attempted to dissolve rather than modify the care of mentally disordered people, sprung up in the 1960s. Perhaps more influential theoretically than practically, anti-psychiatry included such ideologically incompatible figures as the Scottish existentialist-phenomenologist R D Laing (1960), the English Marxist David Cooper (1968), and the American libertarian Thomas Szasz (1972).

Another example of 'alternative' care is the Critical Psychiatry Network (CPNet) whose founders, themselves psychiatrists, claim that they wish to avoid the polarization between traditional psychiatry and anti-psychiatry (Double et al., 2002). They want to have the psychological and social contexts recognized as central to understanding mental disorder rather than just biology, drugs, and coercion. The CPNet highlights the fallibility of relying on a version of science that has capitulated to the randomized control trial, biogenetic aetiology, diagnostic categories, and physical methods of treatment. What is needed is novel dialogue between psychiatrists and service users/survivors whereby both sets of 'expertise' are respected.

But none of the criticisms by the CPNet of psychiatry and science are new or revolutionary, nor is the idea that mentally disordered people should be listened to and understood. What is being championed by the CPNet is an improvement in the mental health system rather than its replacement.

Antagonism towards the formal psychiatric services is active in the UK but disguised in many forms with aims that rarely argue for the dissolution of psychiatry or radical change, but more towards modification. For example, there is the Mental Health Alliance (MHA), formed by scores of pressure groups in 1999, which has campaigned against proposed mental health legislation and the growing numbers of people detained compulsorily. It supports the notion of 'client-centred' care, and users of the mental health services being in charge of their own treatment (Mental Health Alliance, 2002). Such a political position is inherently diametrically opposed to the 'social control' core feature of psychiatric medicine and nursing (Morrall, 1998), but is not advocating the destruction of mental health services as such or that madness is a social construct.

Post-liberalism

The restorative plan has to be 'fitted in' to the Labour Government's overall social democratic political philosophy. New Labour's search for a 'third way' in British politics, which mediates between the individualism of rampant monetarist economics and the social engineering of the 'nanny state', has entered all areas of social policy (Giddens, 1998).

But how 'third wayism' can be translated into mental health and criminal justice policies demands a high level of imagination and political spin-doctoring. Although the changes are presented as a way of avoiding the pitfalls of policies based solely on either the asylum or the community, there is in effect a re-emphasis on institutional care and public safety. That is, the 'third way' gives much more weight to acute in-patient hospital services, secure accommodation, and the need to protect both the public and the mentally disordered by removing 'dangerous' patients from the community, rather than being a pledge to re-invest in the policy of care in the community (Cox, 2002; Warden, 1998a). The Government's 'third way' strategy is best understood within the wider social control context of 'post-liberalism' (Morrall, 2002).

In mature liberal-democracies there has been a major shift in social control measures as a consequence of the fashioning of a new social contract of rights and responsibilities. Denizens becomes citizens. They are expected by the state to be, and they demand of themselves, unprecedented (in modern times) involvement in decision-making within many (if not all) spheres of civil life. They are given the privilege of social inclusion, and have an ethical obligation to participate in the operation of social affairs at the local and national level. No longer will the principles of the free market (no social responsibility, only self-responsibility) or socialism (no self-responsibility, only social responsibility) be the only available political ideologies.

As Nikolas Rose (2000) has suggested, under such socio-political conditions, with an expanding and demanding citizenship, the system of social control has to accommodate and vitalize the active and 'free' subject (through the reward of – apparent – greater freedoms) and denigrate far more robustly (through – very real – harsh punishment) the deviant. Social control in post-liberal society is sophisticated and ubiquitous. It develops as an interwoven pattern of direct and indirect, clandestine and flagrant interventions in daily life – both progressively tolerant (human rights acts, consumer privileges) and at the same time retrogressively despotic (diminution or removal of human rights from some sections of society).

In an epoch where self-regulation is key to social control, those that are perceived (by the state and its semi-detached but synergetic agencies) as failed citizens, spoiled citizens, rebellious citizens, or as members of an underclass of non-citizenship pose an unparalleled threat to civil constancy. They become susceptible to the concomitant discourse of risk thinking, risk management, and the technologies of risk assessment and control. Defaulting on the responsibilies of the new social contract invites demonization. Paedophiles, recidivists (adult criminals, young offenders, prostitutes, drunks, noisy neighbours), the severely mentally ill, and psychopaths – the 'dangerous classes' – are socially or physically confined.

Within the criminal justice sphere, indications of the post-liberal shift include the introduction of: mandatory life-sentences for second serious violent or sexual offences; police registers of sex offenders; electronic 'tagging' of offenders serving community sentences; anti-social behaviour orders aimed at, for example, juvenile miscrants, prostitutes, and disruptive neighbours; neighbourhood wardens and community support officers (proposed) employed to patrol public spaces with powers to deliver fixed penalties and detain suspects; imprisonment for parents of truanting schoolchildren who fail to ensure their children do not truant from school; and a higher profile for victims of crime.

Indications of post-liberalism within the mental health system (some of which overlap with the criminal justice) are: supervision registers for severely mentally ill people living in the community; electronic surveillance, and the increased use of seclusion within psychiatric institutions; 'assertive outreach'; and treatment coercion for community-based patients.

Moreover, the bombing of the World Trade Center in New York on 11 September 2001 has augmented post-liberalism. In the UK, Australia, and the USA emergency legislation has resulted in long-term or indefinite detention without trial or criminal charges for suspected terrorists (Norton-Taylor, 2002).

Terror

Prejudice about mental disorder and social exclusion of the mentally disordered continues (Morrall, 1999), thereby feeding the post-liberal control aspect of mental health policy. Research in which the opinion of young people (500 16–24-year-olds) about mental health found that there was a significant lack of knowledge about the subject (Department of Health, 2001d). Eight out of 10 of the respondents (interviewed by telephone) associated having a mental health problem with discrimination. Over one-half (55%) would not want others to find out that they had a mental health problem. Only one-third of the respondents regarded pejorative language, such as 'schizo', 'loony', 'nutter', and 'psycho', as unacceptable, with nearly two-thirds (61%) themselves using these terms. However, prejudice has spilled over into fear. The overriding influence on 21st century mental health policy in the UK has been an accumulation of media interest, public concern, and criticism from independent inquiries about how the psychiatric disciplines were dealing with the perceived risk from 'dangerous' mad people living in the community.

There is debate about the 'manufacture' or reality of dangerousness and mental disorder (Busfield, 2001). But the consequence of murders by people diagnosed as suffering from mental disorder receiving such media attention, and the apparent lack of rigour by the psychiatric disciplines within the context of a failing health system, has been unequivocally dramatic (Morrall, 2000). It has shifted 'chaos' to 'control'.

Central to this shift is the dispute about how to treat disorders of the personality, and whether some or all forms are even susceptible to treatment (Warden, 1998b). In England, neither the 1983 Mental Health Act nor the 1995 Mental Health (Patients in the Community) Act insist that the psychiatric disciplines have to accept responsibility for those afflicted by a disorder of their personality if they are considered to be 'untreatable'. The case of Michael Stone, diagnosed as suffering from a personality disorder, illustrates the point well. Stone was given three life sentences (and lost his subsequent appeal against the judgment) for the murder of Linda Russell and her six-year-old daughter Megan Russell, and the attempted murder of her other daughter Josie Russell. He had a long history of violent tendencies and had been dealt with previously by the mental health services. Allegedly, he was refused his own request for admission to a psychiatric hospital only days before the crime (Duce and Frean, 1998).

The effect of the Stone case on mental health legislation and policy, and criminal law, has been to encourage the psychiatric disciplines and/or the criminal justice system to embrace a far more proactive stance in dealing with the psychopath. Moreover, this and other similar harrowing incidents pushed the British Government into accepting that there are thousands of people living in the community who are a risk to the public, or will be so on release from prisons and psychiatric institutions.

To curb the freedom of this group – made up of a mixture of child-abusers, rapists, extremely violent individuals, and murderers – a number of proposals have been made by the UK Government. Key professionals (for example, police officers, headteachers, and health and social service work-ers) and community leaders in the area in which the offender is to live on discharge are to be notified of the whereabouts of the dangerous person and of the plans the authorities have for him or her. To follow is the most sensational 'post-liberal' change in the law. People with dangerous severe personality disorder, whether or not they are susceptible to treatment, and pre-emptive of any offence, are to be detained, possibly indefinitely, in accommodation within special hospitals or prisons (Department of Health, 2002d; Home Office and Department of Health, 1999).

Human rights

These post-liberal changes in mental health policy obviously have serious consequences for human rights. In 2000 the UK implemented its first explicit human rights legislation (Human Rights Act 1998: Home Office, 2000) as an albeit belated consequence of the European Convention on Human Rights 1950. The enactment of human rights occurred at a time when widespread community concern, even terror, over the threat from unsupervised mentally disordered people had prompted proposals for increased control (Morrall, 2000). Producing mental health legislation, therefore, has been problematic while case-law unfolds. Certainly, the Mental Health Act 1983 contravenes the Human Rights Act 1998. For example, in a landmark decision a high court judgment has found that the human rights of detained patients were being breached regularly because reviews of the justification for their detention were not taking place quickly enough. The judge reportedly blamed the former Secretary of State for Health, Alan Milburn, for allowing the shortage of mental health review tribunal panel members to occur; the cause of the delays in patients having their cases heard was under-funding from central gov-ernment (Wilson, 2002).

However, human rights protection for the mentally disordered is in any event qualified under this Act (Sainsbury, 2000c). There is the gen-eral principle of 'limited rights', which means that 'persons of unsound mind' can be detained, providing that this is done legally. Another principle of the Act is that of 'qualified rights'. This determines that private life can be interfered with 'for the protection of the rights and freedoms of others'. Removing an individual from his or her home to enforce psychiatric treatment is therefore a possibility if he or she were determined to be a risk to others or him or herself. 'Proportionality' is the third qualifying principle. Here impediment to human rights (for example, the use of restraint or seclusion) is possible on condition that it is not arbitrary or unfair.

On the other hand, a fourth principle is that of 'incompatibility'. All present and future legislation has to be in accord with the Human Rights Act 1998. Given the above caveats, this leaves much scope for the mentally disordered to be regarded as 'excluded' from normal rights protection. Moreover, before a person can be compulsorily detained, a 'true' mental disorder must be established before a 'competent authority' by 'objective' medical experts (Article 5). However, the Act not only omits to define mental disorder in any detail (as occurs in mental health legislation), but also, with further homage to teleology and medical power, posits that the mental disorder must be of a kind or degree warranting compulsory confinement and that the validity of continued confinement depends on the persistence of such a mental disorder. There are also a number of exceptions to these specific conditions (compelled admission can occur in emergencies; discharge may be deferred where there is 'public danger' – although discharge should not be 'unreasonably delayed').

There are no exceptions, however, under Article 3 of the Human Rights Act 1998, which intones that there must be 'freedom from torture and inhuman or degrading treatment or punishment'. The difficulty is that case-law may establish 'therapeutic necessity' as not inhuman or degrading, thereby allowing detention, restraint, seclusion, enforced treatment, and electroconvulsant therapy to continue to be applied as long as it is legal, justified, and transparent.

However, adding to the chaos that is mental health policy, the Royal College of Psychiatrists and the Law Society (2002) have declared that reform of mental health law based on control is 'fundamentally flawed in principle and practice'. They also point out that the new policy is incompatible with the European Convention on Human Rights and therefore the Human Rights Act 1998.

But a resolution might be at hand to resolve this incompatibility. The UK Government, following a lead by the French government, is 'reconsidering its obligations' to European and UK human rights legislation (Verkaik, 2003). Although this reconsideration is targeted at the deportation of 'dangerous' asylum seekers, the focus could be switched to people with 'dangerous' mental disorder.

Experiences

What of the individual's, or his or her carer's, experience within a mental health system characterized by chaos and control?

Magnus Linklater (2001), Chairman of the Scottish Arts Council and a journalist, has written poignantly and lucidly about his encounters with state and private mental health services both in Scotland and England when his son suffered from manic depression (bipolar affective disorder).

> For the past 15 years, my son has suffered from manic depression. I have seen at first hand the shocking deterioration in Britain's mental health services.
>
> (Linklater, 2001: 1)

At the age of 15 years, Linklater's son, Archie, began to deteriorate physically and emotionally. Archie was prescribed antidepressants by a psychiatrist who advised his school. His behaviour, however, was to change dramatically and disturbingly. His language, records his father, became loud, crude, and offensive. After disappearing and being found a day later at a London train station by the police, Archie was placed in a police cell, where he was seen by the school's psychiatrist. Admission to a locked ward in a south London hospital was arranged. Since then, Linklater explains, Archie has had 15 years of 'medical battering' with a range of psychiatric interventions, from elecroconvulsant therapy to cocktails of drugs. For Linklater, this protracted contact with the mental health system has been marked by two experiences. On the one hand, he is grateful to a small group of dedicated doctors and nurses, and for the sensitivity shown by most of the police officers who have dealt with Archie. On the other hand, the appalling circumstances in which such care takes place makes good care extremely difficult: hundreds of unfilled consultant psychiatrist posts resulting in junior doctors taking on responsibilities for which they are ill-trained; filthy and smoke-filled in-patient facilities; a shortage of beds; and inadequate or absent after-care on discharge.

Linklater has received many letters and e-mails from other carers affirming his own view of the inadequacies of mental health provision. For example:

> Although we can tell when our son is becoming hypomanic, there is nothing in the system that allows us to arrange for him to be treated until it is too late. We have no parental rights because he is an adult. As he lives alone there is no one else to care. The police and the health service refuse to deal with him and he will not attend as a voluntary patient when at that stage.
>
> (Communication to Linklater, 2001: 5)

The above account points to the paradox of carers wanting 'control' to be more available when their dependants are at risk to themselves or to others, but either secure and protective environments are not available, or the professionals are unwilling (or unable under the law) to respond to such demands.

Summary

Major reform of the mental health system and more 'ring-fenced' funding is crucial to create calm from chaos. The Sainsbury Centre for Mental Health declares that the two core values of 'equality' (whereby mental disordered people are not discriminated against in such areas of civil life as education, employment, and access to health services) and 'fairness' (those with the greatest need are given the highest priority in health resource allocation) should drive policy (Sainsbury Centre, 2001a). Emerging from these two core values are high quality, comprehensive, and integrated services, which are focused on the needs of the user, and supported by evidence.

However, the overriding influence on 21st century mental health policy in the UK has been an accumulation of media and public attention, and criticism from independent inquiries about how the psychiatric disciplines were dealing with the perceived risk from the 'danger' of mad people living in the community.

Mental health policy in the UK has to be based on a realistic appreciation of the post-liberal agenda of the state, and the role psychiatric medicine and nursing, and associated disciplines (for example, general practice, social work), play within that agenda, i.e. control/hyper-control. The role of the advocacy and lobby agencies (for example, MIND, SANE, Mental Health Alliance) and critics of the mental health system (for example, Critical Psychiatry) becomes one of counterbalance, preventing, as far as possible, excess control and associated human rights abuse. In this sense they are a necessary part of the system they denounce. Emancipation and social integration are feasible only if contact with the formal (and chaotic) mental health services is avoided and the individual relies on his or her social capital and 'hired-help' (for example, private counselling/psychotherapy). However, such emancipation may be the personification of post-liberal self-regulation.

References

Andrews J, Porter R, Tucker P, Waddington K (1997) The History of Bethlem. London: Routledge.

Appleby L (2001) Safety First: Five Year Report of the National Confidential Inquiry into Suicide and Homicide by People with Mental Illness. London: Department of Health.

BBC News (2001) Mental Health Services 'Deteriorating'. http://news.bbc.co.uk/hi/english/health/newsid_1528000/1528376.stm

Beardshaw V, Morgan E (1990) Community Care Works. London: MIND.

Brindle D (1997) Defence budget dwarfed by £32 billion mental health bill. The Guardian, 10 October.

Busfield J (1996) Professionals, the State and the Development of Mental Health Policy. In: Heller T, Reynolds J, Gomm R, Muston R, Pattison S (Eds.) Mental Health Matters: A Reader. Buckingham: Open University Press.

Busfield J (Ed.) (2001) Rethinking the Sociology of Mental Health. Oxford: Blackwell.

Commission for Health Improvement (2002) Clinical Governance Reviews (overview). http://www.chi.nhs.uk/eng/cgr/overview.shtml

Cooper D (1968) Psychiatry and Antipsychiatry. London: Tavistock.

Coppock V, Hopton J (2000) Critical Perspectives on Mental Health. London: Routledge.

Cox J (2002) Mental health: A cultural revolution. PH7 The Parliamentary Health Magazine, 2 (summer): 2.

Department of Health (1998a) Statistics on In-Patients Detained Under the Mental Health Act 1983. Press release (1998/0553). London: Department of Health.

Department of Health (1998b) Modernising Mental Health Services. London: Department of Health.

Department of Health (1999) Mental Health National Service Framework. London: Department of Health.

Department of Health (2000) The NHS Plan: A plan for Investment – A Plan for Reform. London: Stationery Office.

Department of Health (2001a) Mental Health Project. London: Department of Health.

Department of Health (2001b) The National Institute for Mental Health in England: Role and Function. London: Department of Health.

Department of Health (2001c) Mental Health Promotion. London: Department of Health.

Department of Health (2001d) Ignorance and Fear Breeds Negative Mental Health Stigma. http://www.doh.gov.uk/newsdesk/latest/4-nab-12032001.html

Department of Health (2002a) Mental Health Task Force: An Introduction. London: Department of Health.

Department of Health (2002b) Acute In-patient Care Strategy. London: Department of Health.

Department of Health (2002c) National Suicide Prevention Strategy for England Consultation Document. London: Department of Health.

Department of Health (2002d) Draft Mental Health Bill. London: Department of Health.

Double D, Thomas P, Moncrieff J (2002) Critical Psychiatry Network. http://www.critpsynet.freeuk.com/criticalpsychiatry.htm

Duce R, Frean A (1998) Plea for mental help over fantasies of childkilling. The Times, 24 October.

Eastman N (1996) The Need to Change Mental Health Law. In: Heller T, Reynolds J, Gomm R, Mustan R, Pattison S (Eds.) Mental Health Matters: A Reader. Basingstoke: Macmillan/Open University Press. Chapter 24, pp. 205–211.

Fletcher D (1995) Care of mentally ill 'in state of turmoil'. The Electronic Telegraph, 25 August.

Ford R, Durcan G, Warner L, Hardy P, Muijen M (1998) One day survey by the Mental Health Act Commission of acute psychiatric inpatient wards in England and Wales. British Medical Journal, 317: 1279–83.

Gibson M (1999) Reading Witchcraft: Stories of Early English Witches. London: Routledge.

Giddens A (1998) The Third Way. Cambridge: Polity Press.

Gittins D (1998) Madness in its Place: Narratives of Severalls Hospital. London: Routledge.

Goodwin S (1997) Comparative Mental Health Policy. London: Sage

Home Office (2000) Human Rights Act 1998. London: Stationery Office.

Home Office and Department of Health (1999) Managing Dangerous People with Severe Personality Disorder. London: Home Office/Department of Health.

Higgins R, Hurst K, Wistow G (1999) Psychiatric Nursing Revisited: The Care Provided for Acute Psychiatric Patients. London: Whurr.

Institute of Psychiatry (2001) The Maudsley Debates: Plan or Sham? This house believes that the NHS Plan will transform psychiatric care in England for the better. London: Institute of Psychiatry. http://www.iop.kcl.ac.uk/IoP/news/mdebates.stm

Johnstone L (2000) Users and Abusers of Psychiatry: A Critical Look at Traditional Psychiatric Practice. (2nd edition) London: Routledge.

Laing RD (1960) The divided self: An existential study of sanity and madness. London: Tavistock.

Laurance J (2002) The Fear Factory: Mental Health Campaign. The Independent, 30 June.

Laurance J (2003) Pure Madness: How Fear Drives the Mental Health System. London: Routledge.

Linklater M (2001) Bedlam or Asylum. Prospect Magazine, March, http://www.prospect-magazine.co.uk/highlights/witness_linklater_mar01/index.html

MacCabe J (2001) Review – The Maudsley Debates: Plan or Sham? This house believes that the NHS Plan will transform psychiatric care in England for the better. http://www.iop.kcl.ac.uk/IoP/news/mdreview/NHSPlan.html

McCullock A, Muijen M, Harper H (2000) New developments in mental health policy in the United Kingdom. International Journal of Law and Psychiatry, 23 (3–4): 261–76.

Mental Health Alliance (2002) http://www.mind.org.uk/take_action/mha.asp

Milburn A (2003) The NHS needs cultural change [extract from a speech by the Health Secretary to the Social Market Foundation]. The Independent, 1 May.

Miller P, Rose N (Eds.) (1986) The Power of Psychiatry. Cambridge: Polity Press.

Morrall PA (1998) Mental Health Nursing and Social Control. London: Whurr.

Morrall PA (1999) Social Exclusion and Madness: The Complicity of Psychiatric Medicine and Nursing. In: Purdy M and Banks D (Eds.) Health and Social Exclusion. London: Routledge. Chapter 6, pp. 104–21.

Morrall PA (2000) Madness and Murder. London: Whurr.

Morrall PA (2002) Madness, Murder and Social Control. Mental Health Today, August: 23–5.

Morris N (2002) Mental Health Bill is back on the agenda. The Independent, November 15.

National Institute for Clinical Excellence (2002) Schizophrenia: Core Interventions in the Treatment and Management of Schizophrenia in Primary and Secondary Care. London: NICE.

Norton-Taylor R (2002) Terror crackdown 'encourages repression': Human rights responses to September 11. The Guardian, January 17.

Porter R (1987) A Social History of Madness: Stories of the Insane. London: Weidenfeld and Nicolson.

Porter R (2002) Madness: A Brief History. Oxford: Oxford University Press.

Robinson DN (1996) Wild Beasts and Idle Humours: The Insanity Defense from Antiquity to the Present. Cambridge, MS: Harvard University Press.

Rose N (2000) Government and Control. British Journal of Criminology, 40: 321–39.

Royal College of Psychiatrists (2000) Provision of NHS Mental Health Services. Memorandum by the Royal College of Psychiatrists to Select Committee on Health. London: House of Commons Minutes of Evidence (Health: MH 36).

Royal College of Psychiatrists and the Law Society (2002) Reform of the Mental Health Act 1983: Joint Statement by the Royal College of Psychiatrists and the Law Society. http://www.repsych.ac.uk/press/preleases/pr/pr_336.htm

Sainsbury Centre for Mental Health (1997) Pulling Together: The Future Roles and Training of Mental Health Staff. London: Sainsbury Centre.

Sainsbury Centre For Mental Health (1998) Acute Problems: A Survey of the Quality of Care in Acute Psychiatric Wards. London: Sainsbury Centre For Mental Health.

Sainsbury Centre for Mental Health (2000a) The Capable Practitioner. London: Sainsbury Centre for Mental Health.

Sainsbury Centre for Mental Health (2000b) Finding and Keeping: Review of Recruitment and Retention in the Mental Health Workforce. London: Sainsbury Centre for Mental Health.

Sainsbury Centre for Mental Health (2000c) An Executive Briefing on the Implications of the Human Rights Act 1998 for Mental Health Services. London: Sainsbury Centre for Mental Health.

Sainsbury Centre for Mental Health (2001a) Mental Health Policy: The Challenges Facing the New Government. London: Sainsbury Centre for Mental Health.

Sainsbury Centre for Mental Health (2001b) Setting the Standard: The New Agenda for Primary Care Organisations Commissioning Mental Health Services. London: Sainsbury Centre for Mental Health.

Sheppard D (2000) Development of Mental Health Policy and Practice. Institute of Mental Health Law. http://www.imhl.com.history.htm

Standing Nursing and Midwifery Advisory Committee (1999) Mental Health Nursing: Addressing Acute Concern. London: Department of Health.

Szasz TS (1972) The Myth of Mental Illness. Foundations of a Theory of Personal Conduct. St Albans: Paladin.

Thornicroft G (1998) Doing it by halves. The Guardian, February 11.

UKCC (2002) The Recognition, Prevention and Therapeutic Management of Violence in Mental Health Care. London: United Kingdom Central Council for Nursing, Midwifery, and Health Visiting.

Verkaik R (2003) Human Rights in the Balance. The Independent, February 4.

Warden J (1998a) England abandons care in the community for the mentally ill. British Medical Journal, 317 (7173): 1611.

Warden J (1998b) Psychiatrists hit back at home secretary. British Medical Journal, 317 (7168): 1270.

Wilson J (2002) Breach of human rights could start flood of claims by detained patients. The Guardian, April 24.

CHAPTER TWO

US mental health policy: Progress and continuing problems

SHIRLEY A. SMOYAK

Introduction

As the financial cost of mental health care continues to escalate in the USA and other parts of the world, so also does the human cost. It is quite impossible to separate policy, economics, social status markers, education and genetic predispositions into clear areas of scientific or historical inquiry. Access to care is driven not just by policy, but by the resources of patients and families who may find it easy or difficult to get information and weigh decisions. How laws are written and enforced is yet another intersecting domain to be accounted for. They are influenced much more by belief systems and public opinion than by policymakers who consider themselves experts. For instance, although most citizens in the US would embrace the notion that mental and physical health care should be available and accessible to all, 40 million Americans are denied formal access to care (having no health insurance) and the quality of care for others is compromised. It would require another chapter to explain charity care, Medicaid and Medicare and why the proposed Clinton plan for universal health insurance failed.

Another complexity, which needs to be revealed at the outset, is that health professionals, specifically nurses, are now being criticized for not contributing significantly to the public policy debates and formations. Mechanic and Reinhard (2002) have written 'Contributions of Nurses to Health Policy: Challenges and Opportunities'. This article is really titled wrongly, since the points made are that nurses are not doing enough so far as health policy goes. They are not 'coming to the table' and being powerful persuaders to influence policy decisions. This author (Smoyak, 2002c) was invited to write a rejoinder. The main point made is that Mechanic and Reinhard failed to provide 'robust strategies to repair this absence from the inner circles of policy making'. Rather, their advice boils down to 'stop talking only to yourselves and publish in places where you will be noticed'.

The answer to 'Where does the health professional turn when seeking to shape policy?' is a most difficult one (Salmon, 2002). Salmon suggests that nurses are in an opportune position with regard to policy and politics. Nurses are the largest single category of health professional and continue to enjoy the respect and trust of their clients. They are well connected in communities. The great need for the development of skills that support policy development and political action can be met by professional organizations and faculties of nursing rising to the challenge.

Ehrenreich in the same book stridently describes what needs to happen. 'If nursing is to take on a more visionary and activist role, nursing's professional organizations must be willing to back up and support activist nurses who are fired or get into trouble one way or another for their efforts ...' (Ehrenreich, 2002: xxxvi). She ends by addressing those who would criticize such activism, but are profiting from the status quo, and who would say that this is 'not professional behavior (but) troublemaking', with the following. 'I hope that you'll have the determination to answer back: "Well, for the time being, troublemaking is our profession"' (2002: xxxvii).

Comparing the early years in America with the present

An old saying goes, 'The more things change, the more they are the same'. This surely seems to be the case with the care for persons suffering from mental illness in America, and probably is also true for most other developed countries. When America was first settled, and before formal governmental bodies were in place, families and if need be communities were responsible for persons afflicted with mental illness, called lunatics, distracted, or insane. There were no mental health professionals, no hospitals, no scientific theories about the cause of the problem, and no public policy. There was only family care.

Today, families of people with mental illness express feelings of abandonment by health professionals and legislators alike. Not only is hospitalization not usually an option, but also the financial burdens of care fall largely to individuals and families. Just as in colonial times, if the mentally ill family member is not at home, he or she might be in jail, or wandering about as a homeless person, or finding shelter in the modern-day equivalent of poorhouses or almshouses, i.e. residential shelters. The only difference is that the modern patient might occasionally encounter medications, and sources willing to provide them. The other significant differences are that today the illness problems are compounded by the use of substances such as drugs and alcohol, and that patients live longer, thus being more likely to also acquire medical problems (Smoyak, 2000a).

Today the large numbers of psychiatric patients who have been deinstitutionalized, were never institutionalized, or who find themselves in the wrong institutions, such as gaols, are very highly visible. They are of considerable and continued interest: the media, politicians and policymakers, mental health professionals and insurers of all types worry about them and the associated effects on the economy of their care and possible treatment. In contrast, in the 17th and 18th centuries insane persons aroused much less interest. There were no social policies nor governmental provisions for these people. 'Before the American Revolution mental illnesses posed social and economic rather than medical problems' (Grob, 1994: 6–7).

Colonial times and the 19th century

The colonists settling America were strongly influenced by their English traditions and legal practices, yet the reality of the situation in America required dramatically different approaches. As late as 1790, there were just six cities with more than 8,000 residents, which held less than 4% of the entire population. Only two (New York and Philadelphia) had more than 25,000 residents; no city had 50,000. 'Such diffuse populations could not support large institutions to care for the insane' (Grob, 1994: 14).

If the families had sufficient funds, they often built tiny houses or adjacent rooms for their mentally ill members. The accounts of these rooms being only five by seven feet have to be understood in the context that all dwellings were very small. In the 17th century, entire families might occupy one room. The building of a separate space for the ill person was not callous or cruel, but a way to give the family some respite from the behaviour of that person. Communities sometimes subsidized these efforts, if the families were in financial need.

By the early 18th century, growth in the population had increased to the point that institutionalizing disturbing persons was not only considered, but also implemented. At first, the solution was to increase the size of existing almshouses, without making any effort to separate the types of people housed there. As early as 1729, in Boston, the officials built, after gaining quick authorization to do so, a separate place to confine 'distracted persons', apart from the poor (Smoyak, 2000a).

During this period, again borrowing from England, a mixed system of public welfare and private beneficence began to emerge. Hospitals were built by the rich, not for themselves, but for the poor and to train physicians. These philanthropists, building urban hospitals, never intended to use them personally.

By 1850, more than 12 per cent of the population lived in urban settings. In densely populated cities, disturbed and disturbing behaviour was more visible and less tolerated. Family patterns changed, and there were fewer caretakers at home to look after those whose behaviour was problematic. Informal methods of intervening or containing the problems gave way to systematic policies developed by local governments, and then, later, at state levels. Immigration further taxed cities, which were desperately trying to deal with crowding, inadequate housing and increased expenditures for social programmes, such as education and welfare.

Grob makes the point that 'changes in the economy and social structure, however important, could not by themselves have created the mental hospital' (1994: 25). What was required was a drastic shift in thinking, and the willingness to see alternatives to the informal, family-based care. Enlightenment values permeated both Europe and America, replacing the older, fatalistic, deterministic religious teachings about fate and God with a blend of intellectual and scientific currents giving rise to a secular belief that long-standing problems could be solved by conscious and purposeful human intervention.

Along with this new positivism came growing financial support of wealthy elites in urban communities. With the new ideas, new methodologies, and new elites came a growing consensus that government, particularly at the state level, had an obligation to foster the welfare of its citizens. The earlier consensus was that such responsibility rested primarily with cities or local governments. States began to exercise police and regulatory authority to assure that some sort of cohesion prevailed. There was little opposition to the class-based system, which simply reflected the realities of differential wealth and resources evident in all societal sectors. There was no dissent or efforts to reform the situation.

Between the 1840s and 1860s Dorothea Dix led the movement to make public asylums the foundation of public policy (Tiffany, 1890). Dix's dedication to the building of asylums (more than 30) resulted in her also having considerable influence in the sphere of the emerging field of institutional psychiatry. When superintendent positions became vacant, she was consulted for her decisions about replacements. She also mentored younger psychiatrists.

As soon as a state hospital was built, it became full, and then quickly overcrowded. The hospitals became communities apart from the communities in which they were located, since housing was also built for the employees, who stayed on the grounds along with the patients. These 'total institutions', to use Goffman's (1962) term, included dairies, farms, upholstery and dressmaking shops, laundries, bakeries and even delivery rooms. Illegitimate births were not uncommon, since in the crowded dormitories, men and women were not separated. To fight rising costs and reduce boredom, patients worked in the grounds and in the various hospital shops. This was not called 'therapeutic' until decades later and there were no particular policies about these practices.

Legislators had no particular plans for these institutions, other than not to expend more dollars than were actually necessary. There were no long-term plans or policies, since many of the legislators served only one term or very few. There were few permanent staff, and none who stayed long enough to grasp the big picture, or provide an analysis of how the medical, legal, and financing systems were intertwined. There was little or no resistance to public expenditures, and land grants to states to build the hospitals on many acres were very popular.

The attributes of the ideal asylum were specified in a series of propositions adopted by the superintendents in the mid-1850s and further elaborated upon by Thomas S. Kirkbride (1847). His hospital design was referred to as a 'congregate' plan; it specified precisely how rooms were to be arranged, where administrative officers should be placed and so on. The more acute, and more treatable, patients were placed near the front of the hospital. Those not responding to the treatment were moved farther back, in order to make way for new admissions. Much more was written about the physical plant and its arrangement than about either financing or the medical issues. Although state mental hospitals were constantly adding beds and space, they were never adequate to care for all the patients appropriate to be hospitalized.

The issue of who pays for care

States adopted different laws concerning responsibility for the care of disabled or disenfranchised people; these laws varied widely from state to state. In states where the law dictated that local communities were financially responsible for their poor and indigent insane citizens, local officials tended to keep them in local almshouses. In states where the state government assumed the costs, the local officials were very likely to send their citizens to the state asylums.

There were attempts by several leaders, including Dorothea Dix, to shift some of the states' costs to the Federal Government. Each attempt was soundly defeated, sometimes accompanied by impassioned speeches and articles about the hazards of destroying local responsibility and states' rights. It would be another century before the Federal Government became directly involved, by laws and by funding, with the care and treatment of people suffering from mental illness.

Although asylums had not delivered the promises, it would be unfair to overlook their achievements. For many, hospitalization was needed and brought relief at a critical point. Substantial numbers of people were discharged after relatively short stays (three to nine months) and were never re-hospitalized. For those seriously and persistently ill, they provided needed shelter, food and clothing. The fact that chronicity was a considerable facet of mental illness was not noticed nor acknowledged when the political heat insisted that the focus be new methods and cure. Some hospitals discharged patients who did not improve, in order to keep their length of stay statistics in good order. By the 1860s, it was clear that chronicity, as a dimension of insanity, was the single most important issue politically, professionally and financially.

At the turn of the 20th century

One of the most significant changes in the patient population was the absolute number and proportion of persons aged 60 and over. Before 1900, these elderly people with behaviour problems were not committed to asylums, but were cared for at home, unless their behaviour was very life-threatening. Physicians made distinctions between mental disorders in the elderly and non-elderly, reasoning that ageing produced its own special symptoms (forgetfulness, depression, senility, bizarre behaviour) which were simply ageing, and not a psychiatric condition.

Another social factor that influenced how behavioural problems in older persons were handled was that the idea of retirement did not yet exist. People simply worked for as long as they were able, and then relied on family. There was no social security system. Not being able to earn money, particularly for the middle and lower classes, was a very serious problem. When families could not provide for their elders, then the burden of support fell on almshouses, or poorhouses, which had become centrepins in the 19th century welfare system. By the end of the century, however, they were being severely criticized and their utility was in question.

Mental hospitals in the first half of the 20th century changed dramatically in regard to the population served. They became surrogate homes for elderly and other types of chronic cases. There are no national statistics recorded, so the picture had to be pieced together from data gathered by the separate states. New York, for example, offers an especially dramatic picture of change. By 1920, 18% of all first admissions had the diagnosis of either senility or arteriosclerosis. By 1940, this group accounted for one-third of all admissions (Smoyak, 2000b).

To some degree, this outcome occurred not by design, but because of unintended consequences of other changes. In New York, as in other states, the debates had gone on for decades, regarding the appropriate authority for the care and welfare of disenfranchised persons, whether they were poor, elderly or mentally ill. A group of physicians and charity workers formed a coalition, which succeeded in its efforts to have a new law which would end the ambiguity and divide responsibility between local governments and the state. The State Care Act was passed in 1890. The distinction between acute and chronic cases was ended, and all hospitals were placed on an equal footing. A statewide tax to support these institutions was implemented. Local jurisdictions were required to send insane residents to state hospitals; local asylums reverted to poorhouses. Other states quickly followed this new pattern.

As state hospitals turned into huge infirmaries, housing increasing numbers of elderly persons with no acute psychosis, concern was expressed about the cost of such care. The second large group of patients occupying state mental hospitals for whom there was no hope and no cure were those in the tertiary stage of syphilis. There were no antibiotics to treat syphilis in its primary stage before World War II, and so those who reached the third stage suffered severe damage to the central nervous system. Their behaviour was often bizarre and hard to manage; it included seizures, amnesia, delusions, character changes, visual disorders and paralysis.

The large numbers of chronic patients for whom there was no cure produced a very depressing effect on the state hospitals. Attendants and other staff worked in a generally depressed environment, with no ray of hope or positive outcomes in the patients for whom they were responsible. The poor pay and demoralizing work environment produced serious negative behaviours on the part of some staff, who became abusive, mentally and physically, of their patients. Conflict and disorganization were the order of the day (Smoyak, 2000b).

While psychiatrists had been an integral part of the mental hospital system, as the century moved on, they began to disassociate themselves from the hospitals, and seek new domains. After 1900, the new ideology was 'dynamic psychiatry' (as it came to be called), which differed substantially from the 19th century model, which assumed a distinction between health and disease.

In contrast, the new model of psychic distress suggested that behaviour occurred along a continuum, from normal to abnormal, with no demarcation or sharp distinction between states or conditions. Health and disease were now blurred, with theories evolving to pinpoint how environments, or genetics, or other aspects of life histories may colour an individual's response to an internal or external event or challenge. Adolf Meyer was a key figure in American psychiatry from 1890 until his retirement shortly before World War II. Among his major contributions to the field was moving toward a biological and pluralistic view of human beings, and rejecting the kind of dualism implied in the former mind and body distinctions. He insisted that psychiatry had to rest on a 'biologic conception' and reiterated: 'We must ... accept the statement that all mental activity must have its physiological side and its anatomical substratum' (Meyer, 1896).

The belief that it was possible and easier to prevent mental disorders than it was to treat them, once they were full-blown, paved the way for the development of the Mental Hygiene Movement. Actually Clifford Beers, author of *A Mind That Found Itself*, was the instrumental layperson who originated the idea to formalize the movement by developing a national effort to humanize mental hospitals as a first step.

National data on diagnostic categories before 1940 were either imprecise or non-existent. Yet, using a variety of estimation and approximation methods, the fact that the overwhelming majority of patients had a severe mental illness diagnosis was clear. Demographic data provided a further perspective. The US Census Bureau data from 1910 found that 63.5% of the male in-patient population was single, 6.6% widowed or divorced, and 26.4% married. For women, comparable percentages were 41.7, 15.7, and 40.4. By contrast, in the general population, 55.8% of males and 58.9% of females were married. Of the in-patient population, about 69% were over 40 years old. Clearly, the majority of mentally ill persons hospitalized did not have either spouses or parents available to provide care for them. There were no community support systems in place. No wonder, then, that the hospital system remained in place, while serious attacks on it were a constant reality.

Mid-20th century and World War II

The deplorable conditions in state hospitals during the war were documented in newspaper articles and professional journals. Dorothy Deming, a nurse employed by the American Public Health Nurses' Association, noted critical shortages in many states. One hospital with 6,000 patients had 168 attendants on duty, compared with the normal complement of 538. Such news was not disseminated widely: the media were not yet interested in these problems. No nationwide journal for psychiatric nurses existed until two decades later. Data about nurses appear in the context of studies about other personnel. For instance, an independent survey by the Group for the Advancement of Psychiatry post-WW II found serious shortages of physicians and nurses. Overcrowding reached 74% in some settings. In one hospital, the doctor–patient ratio was 1:500, while the nurse–patient ratio was 1:1,320 (Smoyak, 2000c).

While the energies and resources of the nation for the most part were occupied by war during the 1940s, several major somatic therapies were introduced into the state hospital system, most having their origins in Europe. Fever, metrazol, insulin and electric shock therapy, and lobotomies, were performed in almost all of the larger hospitals. Hospital records showed no comparisons of expenses, or justification for their continued use by any scientific evaluative method. Although hospitals were dramatically under-staffed, these treatments were given, with little consideration of documentation or aftercare. For instance, while nurses certainly must have participated in these treatments and been concerned with their *ad hoc* nature, the *American Journal of Nursing* carried no opposing clinical or questioning articles about such practices. In Smoyak and Rouslin's (1982) *A Collection of Classics in Psychiatric Nursing Literature*, a letter is printed from an associate editor of the *American Journal of Nursing*, rejecting a psychiatric nursing article, and explaining that while the article was outstanding, the journal was not 'in the market' for another one at the time (1942) because one had just been printed last year (Smoyak, 1982: 7).

In Gerald Grob's lectures about the historical aspects of the care of mental patients, he often returns to the issue of 'unintended consequences' in the course of life and policymaking. World War II had far-reaching unintended consequences for how care would be delivered to people with mental illnesses. During this war, military psychiatrists found that neuropsychiatric disorders were far more pervasive and serious than had been previously recognized. The psychiatrists were convinced that environmental stress associated with combat leads to mental maladjustment, and that early treatment in noninstitutional settings produces favourable outcomes. These conclusions were reached, not as a result of any controlled studies, but from clinical observations of the pragmatic approaches applied. The psychiatric casualties were removed from the war zone, and treated locally (at the company aid station level), not further back (such as rear echelon units) or returned home. The treatment was largely supplying respite from battle and providing basic requirements such as showers, beds and food.

From these successes, the psychiatrists logically concluded that treatment in civilian life could be organized the same way, provided in a family/community setting rather than in some remote, isolated institution. Much energy was spent convincing politicians and policymakers that this was an accurate assessment. The psychiatrists themselves planned to work at the community level rather than in institutions when the war ended.

The military psychiatrists returned after the war, and set out to convince Congress that immediate action needed to be taken to institute new treatment approaches, based on their war experiences. They advocated an end to asylum methods, and putting in place an alternative method, which included early identification of symptoms and treatment in community settings. As one measure of their persuasive success, Congress passed and President Truman signed into law the National Mental Health Act in 1946.

Three basic goals were incorporated in the National Mental Health Act: (1) to support research relating to the cause, diagnosis and treatment of psychiatric disorders; (2) to train mental health personnel by providing individual fellowships and institutional grants; and (3) to award grants to states to assist in the establishment of clinics and treatment centres and to fund demonstration projects dealing with the prevention, diagnosis and treatment of neuropsychiatric disorders. It also created a National Mental Health Advisory Council and established the National Institute for Mental Health (NIMH).

During the 1950s, community-oriented and prevention programmes were developed in every state, although they varied considerably in their funding, direction, and staffing patterns. Ironically, with all the enthusiasm and positive speech-making about the community psychiatric movement, and the successes of NIMH, there were no guidelines or protocols for personnel, for training, or for evaluation of the various new programmes. There were no policies in place; rather, the directions taken were largely pragmatic.

During the 1950s, other developments served to shape the field, the politics and the funding patterns. Psychotropic drugs and milieu therapy were introduced almost simultaneously, and described as entities which would definitely prepare hospitalized patients for discharge to communities. Electroshock and psychosurgery were still prevalent. The new schools of psychotherapy were developing rapidly. The costs for these new therapies were covered differentially, depending on the setting. Psychotherapy was largely practised on an out-patient basis, and paid for in fee-for-service arrangements. At first, insurance companies paid the bill. In the public hospitals, staff from all the mental health disciplines learned the new 'group work' skills, with psychotherapeutic underpinnings, and the cost was folded into staff salaries, and never accounted for as a separate item.

Chlorpromazine was the first antipsychotic drug to be introduced in the mid-1950s. Smith Kline and French (SKF), its developers, saw the field of psychiatric nursing as a valuable ally in getting the message across that Thorazine (SKF's trade name for chlorpromazine) would be an asset in preparing patients for psychotherapeutic approaches to their treatment and eventual discharge. SKF financially underwrote the production of the classic film, *The Nurse–Patient Relationship*, which featured the work of the psychiatric nursing pioneer, Hildegard E. Peplau. SKF paid film writers to sit in Peplau's seminars at Greystone Park Psychiatric Hospital in New Jersey. After they produced the script, approved by Peplau, the filming was done on wards at the hospital, with student nurses and staff posing as patients. The cost of the film and its distribution was accounted for within the marketing domain. Other such efforts include the famous 'purple pamphlet' where the highlights of Peplau's work in teaching interviewing techniques and psychotherapy were captured (Smoyak, 2000c).

After prolonged debate and discussion between the American Medical Association and the American Psychiatric Association in the mid-1950s, they agreed to sponsor a joint commission with two goals: (1) to inventory all resources and methods employed in the diagnosis, care and treatment of the mentally ill and mentally retarded, and (2) to formulate a feasible programme of improvement. Although the Joint Commission on Mental Illness and Health (JCMIH) would be sponsored by the two professional groups, Congress passed the Mental Health Study Act, which paved the way for modest federal funding.

In summary, what the report recommended was a doubling of expenditure for public mental health patient services in five years, and a tripling in 10 years. Obviously such an investment could only be met by a massive increase in federal funding. At the end of 10 years, the federal share of costs would be 58% of all mental health expenditures and states would pay 33%, while the cost share for local units would be 9%. The press release for Action for Mental Health embodied a perhaps exaggerated – although not entirely unrealistic – feeling, when it suggested, that, if the Joint Commission's recommendations became law, this would 'revolutionize public care of persons with major mental illness – the nearly 1 million patients who pass through state hospitals and community mental health clinics each year' (JCMIH Press Release, 1961).

The last 50 years

In December 1961, President Kennedy created an Interagency Task Force on Mental Health. Albert Ribicoff, Secretary of Health, Education and Welfare, was the nominal chair, but the actual work was done by a group that included Robert Felix, Stanley Yolles (Felix's deputy), and Daniel Patrick Moynihan. At the same time, NIMH appointed its own internal groups to formulate policy recommendations. The first NIMH group criticized state hospitals on the grounds that they fostered dependency and were burdened by archaic administrative systems. The second believed that the community-oriented approach was the way for the future to be shaped.

Under President Johnson, the Great Society programmes were in tune with community psychiatry and the community mental health centres (CMHCs). Funds for construction and staffing, however, declined as the Vietnam War escalated. The gap between authorization and funding widened each year. By 1980, the total number of CMHCs was 754, far short of the original goal of 2,000.

CMHCs were not serving the patients leaving the state hospitals, but rather developing a very different population base that was not seriously mentally ill. Many centres emphasized programmes for children and adolescents, for divorcing families, or for other types of problems not at all in the range of psychotic populations. Their funding was not affected by the failure to provide active outreach or programming for patients discharged from state hospitals. In fact, very few did any type of outreach or considered diagnoses such as schizophrenia to be their main mission.

Another 'unintended consequence' of federal policy was the passage of amendments to the Social Security Act of 1935. Congress, in 1965, with Presidential approval and prodding, passed a series of amendments which would have profound effects on the financing of care for persons seriously mentally ill. Medicare and Medicaid were designed to provide medical care for the aged and the poor. Title 18, Part A (Medicare) was the hospital insurance part for persons over 65; Part B paid for physicians' services. Title 19 (Medicaid) involved grants to states for medical assistance programmes for indigent persons. Surprisingly, psychiatric benefits were included. The public often thinks of Medicaid as a source of help for mothers and children needing welfare, but persons with mental illness are also included. Medicaid became an important source of funding for elderly persons in mental hospitals, although payments were limited. The limitation on the use of Medicare and Medicaid funds for aged persons in state hospitals produced a dramatic shifting of people. States acted to curtail their costs by sending such patients from the state hospitals to nursing homes, because the latter benefited by far more generous federal payments for this category.

The unintended consequence of Titles 18 and 19 was a massive shifting of patients from hospitals to nursing homes, if they were over 65. The discharge of patients from the hospitals was called 'deinstitutionalization', but in fact was more accurately 'transinstitutionalization'. When considering the younger patients who were discharged with inadequate community supports, the 'transinstitutionalization' which occurred found them in gaols. In many ways, these moves mirrored the shifts of patients from almshouses to hospitals and back again, or to the street.

In 1975, Congress passed a new mental health law, which increased the mandated essential services from five to 12. They included follow-up services and programmes for the elderly, as well as alcohol and drug abuse problems. In just five years another new Mental Health Systems Act was passed, with Rosalynn Carter playing a major role. It assumed continued federal leadership, even though the CMHCs would eventually lose all federal support. The ink was hardly dry on this new law, when it and its provisions became moot. President Reagan immediately reversed all policy just put in place, and focused his energies on reducing both taxes and federal expenditures. Federal funds were cut by 25% and Federal mental health programmes were shifted into block grants to states. This move completely reversed the earlier Federal ideology that a strong central administration was necessary to bring some degree of conformity and basic quality to state programmes.

By the summer of 1981, the Omnibus Budget Reconciliation Act was signed into law. It provided for block grants to states for mental health services and substance abuse, and repealed most of the provisions of the Mental Health Systems Act. In the next decade, the focus of policy and funding shifted responsibility back to the states and local communities, coming full circle to the way things were before World War II. In earlier centuries, such massive policy changes occurred only in a matter of decades. In the last decades of this century, significant changes occurred with each new administration, and often within the actual terms of office. Just as the Federal Government had decided to go 'out of business' in matters of mental health policy, authority and funding, states were faced with new social crises and demands for increases in welfare.

Mental health benefits have vastly expanded under private, nonprofit and government insurance programmes, despite continuing disagreements about what mental illness is; how, when and where to treat it; who the providers should be and how they should be trained, and how proportionately responsible the Federal, state and local governments should be. The most recent information about benefits in health insurance plans comes from surveys by the Bureau of Labor Statistics and the Department of Labor. Most people who have insurance policies that cover mental health and substance abuse find that they have severe restrictions compared with medical diagnoses.

There is huge controversy about how the various managed care plans have had an impact on how care is rationed or actually delivered. In the past, indemnity insurers relied on the professional to determine the service or treatment needed, and paid the bill. Mechanic points out that:

> Increasingly, however, managed care companies through HMOs (Health Maintenance Organizations) and utilization review seek to be more precise about what conditions should be treated and about the length and types of treatments that are medically necessary. Treatment for diagnoses not covered by DSM (Diagnostic and Statistical Manual of Mental Disorders) are unlikely to be covered ...
>
> (Mechanic, 1999: 129)

Much effort is expended in avoiding in-patient admissions, reducing in-patient stays, and truncating long courses of treatment. Whenever and wherever possible, managed care requires alternative treatments that are less intensive and less costly. Brief sessions of psychotherapy have replaced the lengthy former model. Psychotropic drugs are ordered as a first choice, often without psychotherapy.

Advanced practice psychiatric nurses, especially those with prescriptive authority, are now included in many of the managed care panels. On the one hand, this can be viewed as an advancement professionally, and hailed as an enlightenment of the insurers. On the other hand, the primary reason for their increased inclusion at this point in time is that they cost less than psychiatrists do. When master's-prepared psychiatric nurses could provide only psychotherapy, in one of its models or schools, they were no different than social workers or psychologists. Now all 50 states have changed their practice laws to include prescriptive authority for nurses.

There is great variability in terms of the level of their independence in prescribing and monitoring their patients' progress.

Both nurses and psychiatrists, as well as general practitioners, who treat persons with mental illness will no doubt continue to complain about how the managed care organizations interfere with their clinical judgement. For instance, the managed care deciders intervene in prescribing practices by insisting that less powerful, less costly, generic (where possible) medications are ordered. Also, they demand that clinicians justify long-term use of medications, and try to introduce protocols whereby there are attempts to wean the patients from the drugs, or stop them entirely. Mechanic describes this new state of affairs very succinctly:

> It seems clear that healthcare system changes are altering mental health practices in significant ways, limiting the autonomy and discretion of clinicians, changing the balance between clinical judgment and administrative expectations, and introducing and applying practice guidelines to the treatment of specific conditions.
>
> (Mechanic, 1999: 129)

Ironically, without the passage of any new laws, and without debate and discussion among professional mental health practitioners, practice patterns are being significantly changed. The changes that are qualitative are sometimes harder to discern than the more visible quantitative ones, such as limiting days of service, or increasing copayments. Protocols and guidelines for providing treatments for specific illnesses are being constructed by the managed care companies. Sometimes the first clue that a professional person will have that change has occurred is when payment for treatments formerly reimbursed are now curtailed. More commonly, the prior approval mechanism comes into play, even when providers have been on panels before. Insurance companies and managed care reviewers have usurped the authority to decide what is clinically necessary, and are defining the dimensions of what appropriate treatment is.

Along with market expansion came some highly unethical practices, and lawsuits against private psychiatric hospitals, that drew the attention of the general public. In 1994, Sally McDonald's article about her deciding to speak up about an unethical practice she was seeing repeatedly at the private psychiatric hospital where she was employed as a registered nurse appeared in the *Journal of Psychosocial Nursing and Mental Health Services*; this created repercussions for her (McDonald, 1994), which resulted in her losing her job. In a follow-up article, A Whistle-Blowing Retrospective (McDonald, 1999), she describes its use as a reference point for three subsequent lawsuits. As in earlier times, when psychiatric nurses witnessed abuses in asylums, they did not engage in any advocacy actions; present-day psychiatric nurses seem reluctant to act as well.

While beds in the private sector expanded, public hospitals continued to try to reduce their size, or at least to both step up discharge processes and ward off new admissions. The present population in most states consists of younger, sicker, harder-to-handle patients than a decade ago. Ironically, the private sector is still organized along business lines, and developing profitable programmes. For-profit development in in-patient psychiatric centres concentrates on affective disorders, substance abuse, adjustment disorders, and even obesity. Hospitals are built in states that have more favourable regulations and less competition. They tend to discharge patients when their insurance benefits have been expended. The patients either return home, or seek admission in the public sector.

Policymaking for people with mental illness is a very difficult process, since the sociocultural, environmental, and even geographic factors weigh so heavily in how the illness is experienced and understood, and how life experiences shape what is believed to be the best approach to care and treatment. Policies that address parity are indeed needed, but are only one piece of a very complex and convoluted problem. To add to the complexity of measuring the outcomes of service, the patient and provider, by the nature of the interchange, create a new social unit. Whether or not there is consensus about the presenting problem, the proposed solution certainly affects outcomes.

A new policy idea: Integrating mental health in primary health

Americans like convenience, and they like to have what they need or want instantly. In the USA, they have grouped materials and services in interesting ways. For instance, they can fill cars with gasoline and fill themselves with coffee and a doughnut at the same time. Banks used to have one focus per institution; now there is one-stop banking in most urban settings, where chequing, saving, mortgaging and getting a loan can happen in one visit. Grocery stores have become mini-malls and include pharmacies (with blood-pressure checking devices), flower shops and photography centres.

The associated new belief is that providing good healthcare requires that it also be integrated. The advent of primary care a quarter of a century ago was heralded as the way to assure accessible, affordable, appropriate services. Fragmentation was supposed to end when practitioners adopted the new ways of organizing care. The associated frustrations with various barriers to care were supposed to become history.

Ironically, parallel to this new interest in providing one-stop shopping for patients, the old fragmentation and animosity between nurses and physicians continued. The nursing shortage of the 1960s had multiple causes. The National Commission for the Study of Nursing and Nursing Education identified professional problems in the workplace as key reasons for nurses leaving their positions. The perceived low status of nurses and associated low salaries accounted for difficulties in enticing new recruits to nursing. As Jerry Lysaught pointed out in *Abstract for Action* (1971) and *From Abstract into Action* (1973) nurses were fed up with the doctor–nurse game and distressed enough with the bossiness and belligerence of physicians that they left nursing.

The American Medical Association (AMA) and the American Nurses' Association (ANA) acted on one of Lysaught's recommendations and brought together eight physicians and eight nurses to construct and implement a plan for ending interprofessional conflicts. The tensions between the two professions were seen as root causes of the inability to implement primary care. The AMA and ANA appointees developed the National Joint Practice Commission (NJPC), which attempted by various strategies during the 1970s to integrate the work of the two professions (Hoekelman, 1974; Smoyak, 1977). Since the AMA did not think that psychiatrists were really physicians, there was no psychiatrist appointed.

Now, 25 years later, working on integrating mental health in primary health has become a policy direction. Surgeon General David Satcher convened a meeting in late 2000 'to advance the integration of mental health services and primary healthcare'. This meeting was an outgrowth of the 1999 Surgeon General's Report on Mental Health. A nurse, Brenda Reiss-Brennan, MS, APRN, CS, and President of Primary Care Family Therapy Clinics, served as the consultant and meeting organizer, conducting over 90 interviews in preparation for the deliberations among the participants representing healthcare professionals, consumers, families, foundations and government agencies. Included among the interviewees were experts representing businesses, researchers, employers, economists, epidemiologists, providers, healthcare consultants and payors, as well as the participants listed above.

Among the group's recommendations were the following:

1. Convene a group under the auspices of the DHHS to develop a framework for the integration of mental healthcare and primary care, including a focus on comorbidities, diverse modalities, and diverse populations. (Note: This is very similar to the mission of the NJPC, but including mental health.)
2. Incorporate a list of skills, knowledges, attitudes, and simple tools that reflects evidence-based 'best practices' and treatment management, leading to improved outcomes. (Note: The providers of such services are not named. The NJPC's idea of 'those who learn together earn together' might yet be a reality.)
3. Design education and training standards for the integration of mental healthcare and primary care with all stakeholders, including accreditation bodies and promote implementation of those standards by schools of health and behavioural health (Smoyak, 2002a).

Psychiatric nurses: Present-day data

The new *Mental Health, United States, 2000,* just released by the US Department of Health and Human Services, shows that psychiatric nurses are a minority in the mental health field. The 15,330 master's-prepared psychiatric nurses are a tiny group, compared with 40,731 psychiatrists, 77,456 psychologists, 31,278 school psychologists, 96,407 social workers and 44,225 marriage and family therapists. Perhaps the most startling statistic is that there are now 100,000 professionals with master's degrees in psychosocial rehabilitation. This group is the newest addition to the ranks of mental health professionals and is graduating a significant number of people. Counsellors, also a relatively new group to the field, but also licensed, number 108,104.

This new volume is very different from its predecessors, with three new sections appearing before the familiar update on the national statistics for mental health. The first section presents an editorial prospective written by Manderscheid and Henderson. They have constructed four scenarios to examine changes in the roles that people with mental illness will be playing in the future. Professionals from all disciplines will need to learn how to collaborate fully with people for whom they are offering care. Frances Hughes, a Commonwealth Fellow (2002), has also forecast this projected change. She adds a Type III to the practice models identified by the National Joint Practice Commission in the 1970s (Smoyak, 1977). Type I describes work that is highly specific, with practitioners undergoing rigorous training for the specialty. Type II work can be accomplished by generalist practitioners from different backgrounds. Type III work is accomplished in a collaborative mode, with patients and practitioners sharing in the assessment and decision making about treatment strategies.

In the second section, four chapters assess the status of mental health statistics at the millennium. 'Decision Support 2000+' is a new information system for mental health which promises to bring updated data accurately and swiftly to the table for use by researchers, practitioners and administrators. The information needs of consumers and families are described. Advances in psychiatric epidemiology as well as accountability efforts are included.

The data presented reflect information only on nurses with graduate degrees in psychiatric/mental health nursing. Many psychiatric nurses, however, have less than master's degrees and can be found in hospital and community settings. Such is the case in clinical settings across the country. It is impossible to produce an accurate accounting of the educational background and post-graduation training for the nurses in psychiatric settings who had their basic preparation in diploma, associate degree or baccalaureate degree programmes. The good news is that in the actual clinical settings, a spirit of collegiality and team building is the case in most instances. Clinical specialists and the newer psychiatric nurse practitioners serve as mentors and guides for the other nurses (Smoyak, 2002b).

Issues and debates about certification mechanisms and boards continue. The current three types of preparation, Clinical Nurse Specialist, Nurse Practitioner, and combined, present dilemmas for those who write the certification examinations. Further, while other disciplines/professions reserve certification processes for those with advanced preparation, nursing has muddied the waters considerably by certifying generalists.

Future directions

As consumers become stronger advocates for themselves, and are joined by family members and professionals who value accountability, the outcome will surely be closer scrutiny about how practices are conducted. The bottom line will be: Are things better for the client? Ways to measure outcomes in psychiatric practice, when the consumer–professional relationship is the focus, need to be developed. When consumers and nurses are equally knowledgeable about medications, side-effects, alternative approaches to therapy, the value of dialogue, and action-oriented treatment, mental illness will surely lose considerable stigma. Nurses and consumers will enjoy new respect at work and in communities. It would be wonderful to 'hurry' this future (Smoyak, 2002b).

References

Ehrenreich B (2002) The emergence of nursing as a political force. In Mason D, Leavitt J, Chaffee M (Eds.) Policy and Politics in Nursing and Health Care, 4th Edition. St. Louis, MO: Saunders.

Goffman E (1962) Asylums: Essays on the Social Situation of Mental Patients and other Inmates. New York: Doubleday.

Grob G (1994) The Mad Among Us: A History of the Care of America's Mentally Ill. New York: The Free Press.

Hoekelman R (1974) Nurse–Physician Relationships: Problems and Solutions. Commencement address to graduates of the Pediatric and Medical Nurse Associate Training Programs, Rush-Presbyterian, St. Luke's Medical Center, Chicago, Illinois, June 26.

Hughes F (2002) Healthcare Delivery Issues: Key Lessons from the United States. Paper prepared for the Commonwealth Fund, Harkness Fellowship, April, 2002 at the University of Pennsylvania, Philadelphia, PA.

JCMIH (1961) Press Release, March 24. In RL Robinson File Action for Mental Health, Box 6, JCMIH Papers, quoted by Grob, 1994: 248.

Kirkbride T (1847) On the construction and arrangements of hospitals for the insane. American Journal of the Medical Sciences, 13: 40–56.

Lysaught J and National Commission for the Study of Nursing and Nursing Education (1971) Abstract for Action. New York: McGraw Hill.

Lysaught J and National Commission for the Study of Nursing and Nursing Education (1973) From Abstract to Action. New York: McGraw Hill.

Mechanic D (1999) Mental Health and Social Policy: The Emergence of Managed Care. Boston: Allyn and Bacon.

Mechanic D, Reinhard S (2002) Contributions of nurses to health policy: Challenges and opportunities. Nursing and Health Policy Review, 1(1): 7–15.

Meyer A (1896) A short sketch of the problems of psychiatry. American Journal of Insanity 53. In Winters E (Ed.) The Collected Papers of Adolf Meyer. 4 volumes. Baltimore, MD, 1950–1952.

McDonald S (1994) An ethical dilemma: Risk and responsibility. Journal of Psychosocial Nursing and Mental Health Services, 32(1): 19–25.

McDonald S (1999) A whistle-blowing retrospective. Journal of Psychosocial Nursing and Mental Health Services, 40(1): 14–27.

Salmon M (2002) Forward. In Mason D, Leavitt J, Chaffee M (Eds.) Policy and Politics in Nursing and Health Care, 4th Edition. St. Louis, MO: Saunders.

Smoyak, S (1977) Problems in interprofessional relationships. Bulletin of the New York Academy of Medicine 53(1): 51–9.

Smoyak S (2000a) The history, economics and financing of mental health care. Part I, 17th to 19th Centuries. Journal of Psychosocial Nursing and Mental Health Services 38(9): 26–33.

Smoyak S (2000b) The history, economics and financing of mental health care. Part II, the 20th Century. Journal of Psychosocial Nursing and Mental Health Services, 38(10): 26–37.

Smoyak S (2000c) The history, economics and financing of mental health care. Part III, The Present. Journal of Psychosocial Nursing and Mental Health Services, 38(10): 26–37.

Smoyak S (2002a) Integrating mental health and primary health. Journal of Psychosocial Nursing and Mental Health Services, 40(4).

Smoyak S (2002b) Psychiatric nursing: A minority mental health profession. Journal of Psychosocial Nursing and Mental Health Services, 40(5): 6–7.

Smoyak S (2002c) Rejoinder to Mechanic and Reinhard. Nursing and Health Policy Review. In press.

Smoyak S, Rouslin S (Eds.) (1982) A Collection of Classics in Psychiatric Nursing Literature. Thorofare, NJ: Charles B. Slack.

Tiffany F (1890) Life of Dorothea Lynde Dix. Boston: Riverside Press.

CHAPTER THREE

Human rights, citizenship and mental health reform in Australia

MIKE HAZELTON AND MICHAEL CLINTON

Introduction

Australia is a highly industrialized liberal-democratic nation with a population approaching 20 million. Colonization by people from Great Britain and subsequently other countries commenced in 1788, resulting in an ethnically diverse present-day society in which 23% of residents were born overseas. Indigenous Australians, known as Aboriginal peoples and Torres Strait Islanders, comprise 2% of the total population. Average life expectancy at birth is 81.5 years for females and 75.9 years for males. On average the life expectancy of indigenous Australians is approximately 20 years less than other Australians (Australian Institute of Health and Welfare, 2000). The country has a federated system of government with six states and two territories (Whiteford et al., 2000).

Recent estimations suggest that about one million Australians suffer from a mental problem or disorder. Although more than half of these are affected long term, a much smaller proportion will seek help or receive a diagnosis for their problem (Australian Institute of Health and Welfare, 2000: 76). Thus while a large number of Australians are affected by mental illness, the full extent of unmet need for treatment has only recently become apparent (Andrews and Henderson, 2000; Jablensky et al., 2000).

In Australia, mental health services are provided in both institutional and community settings. Psychiatric hospitals and psychiatric wards in acute hospitals provide specialized psychiatric care. Community-based mental health services provide assessment, crisis intervention, case management and rehabilitation. Residential facilities provide round-the-clock care and support in the community, and the non-government sector provides supported accommodation and advocacy services. Specialist forensic, early psychosis, dual diagnosis, child and adolescent, and dementia specific services have been developed and implemented. General practitioners also make an important contribution to the care of many Australians with mental illness (Australian Institute of Health and

43

Welfare, 2000). A recent initiative of the Commonwealth Government is to permit general practitioners to provide structured psychological treatment to people with a mental health problem or disorder on a fee-for-service basis. Alternatively, the general practitioner may choose to contract an allied health professional, psychologist, mental health nurse, or occupational therapist to provide these services as part of a treatment plan negotiated with the patient.

Mental health has recently been identified as a National Health Priority Area in Australia (Commonwealth Department of Health and Aged Care and Australian Institute of Health and Welfare, 1999) and in the last decade the country's mental health services have undergone sweeping reforms which have placed them in the forefront of a global transition from predominantly institutional to predominantly community-based care for people with mental problems and disorders (Jablensky et al., 2000: 222). The reforms have been co-ordinated through a National Mental Health Strategy, which has been put into effect through successive five-year implementation plans.

Nevertheless, despite significant improvements in areas such as expenditure and the mix of in-patient and community services, concern continues to be expressed that the shift from institutional to community treatment 'has not delivered the social integration of mentally ill persons anticipated by the ideologies of the community mental health movement' (Coffey, 1994: 32). To date progress in combating discrimination and safeguarding the rights of those with mental illness has lagged behind other key policy areas. There has been little impact on what Johnstone (2001: 202) has referred to as 'culturally normative prejudice' and it has been argued that health professionals often display the most unfavourable attitudes towards the mentally ill (Deakin Human Services Australia, 1999; Johnstone, 2001). Moreover, the implications of deinstitutionalization for community services such as rehabilitation, housing, employment and community support have not been fully appreciated, and this has increased the burden faced by the families of the mentally ill (Deakin Human Services Australia, 1999: 11; Human Rights and Equal Opportunity Commission, 1993). Despite a decade of reform, it is not clear that there have been substantial improvements to the life circumstances of those with mental illness.

This chapter examines what has been achieved after a decade of reform under Australia's National Mental Health Strategy, with particular reference to issues surrounding the protection of human rights and access to the entitlements of citizenship. The next section provides a brief historical outline of the development of mental health services in Australia. This is followed by an overview of the National Mental Health Strategy up to the end of the second five-year implementation plan. Attention then shifts to a discussion of the prospects for achieving the human rights and citizenship reforms that are so central to policy developments in this area.

Historical background

In the early decades following the establishment of the new colony at Sydney Cove, 'treatment' for insanity, when this was available, sometimes included incarceration in a 'safe place'. When the local gaols, which were used initially for this purpose, were found to be unsuitable, special asylums were established under state authority (Crichton, 1990). The asylums of the colonial period have been characterized as providing a 'controlled and sheltered' life for the residents (McDonald, 1983: 189). It was expected that within the high walls and barred windows the daily regimen would revolve around 'cleanliness, kindness, nutrition, medical attention, recreation and good record keeping' (Human Rights and Equal Opportunity Commission, 1993: 4). In New South Wales, the appointment of F Norton Manning to oversee mental health facilities in 1868 saw the beginning of a period of consolidation and expansion. Following a visit to the UK Manning moved to introduce moral treatment into the colonial asylums. New institutions were built and management processes were upgraded in a programme of reforms that set the template for mental health services in New South Wales, and to some extent in other states, until well into the 20th century (Crichton, 1990: 21).

In the decades prior to and following World War I, the development of mental health services was seriously affected by a shortage of funds (Crichton, 1990: 32). This trend continued throughout the years of the Great Depression and World War II so that by the mid-1950s a national inquiry into mental health services (Stoller and Arscott, 1955) was able to conclude that long-term official neglect had contributed significantly to a situation in which Australian mental health services had failed to keep pace with comparable services overseas (Dax, 1975; Lewis, 1988).

At the same time, however, the post-war decades also saw an increase in social pressure for reform. In response to developments in psychiatric treatment, population growth and increasing concern over the costs of maintaining ageing institutions, questions began to be raised regarding the efficacy of the asylum system. There was a growing consensus that the advantages offered by the asylums 'were outstripped by the disadvantages of confinement, exclusion, stigmatization, overcrowding and lack of personal freedom' (Human Rights and Equal Opportunity Commission, 1993: 136). By the 1960s a mental health community-care movement was emerging, as developments in both social psychiatry and psychopharmacology promised the possibility of managing even severely mentally ill patients in the community.

While it has been suggested that much of the impetus for reform was provided by mental health professionals and governments (Lewis, 1988), there is no doubt that a series of controversies over the mistreatment of patients played an important part in shaping the public agenda on mental health reform (Coffey, 1994). Thus from the 1970s onwards, when policymakers spoke of the 'normalization' of residents in mental institutions, and treatment using the 'least restrictive alternative' (Crichton, 1990: 104), they often did so in the context of 'managing' allegations surrounding the abuse of patients in mental health services. Indeed, in New South Wales alone, approximately 40 inquiries were conducted into psychiatric facilities and services between the early decades of the colonial period and the end of the 1980s (Human Rights and Equal opportunity Commission, 1993: 5).

By the late 1970s and 1980s, in many locations throughout the country, community-based mental health services were developing as psychiatric institutions were being allowed to run down. Between the early 1960s and the early 1990s the transition from institutional-based care to community-based care saw a decline in the availability of psychiatric beds, from 281 beds per 100,000 population to 40 beds per 100,000 (Australian Institute of Health and Welfare, 2000: 316–7). However, these developments were often uneven and unco-ordinated within and across state and territory jurisdictions, and resources were typically insufficient to sustain the growth of comprehensive community-based mental health services (Coffey, 1994: 32). In a major inquiry conducted in the early 1990s, the Human Rights and Equal Opportunity Commission (1993: 3) asserted that governments had largely failed to provide sufficient resources to protect the fundamental rights of those with mental illness.

The period of the 1970s and 1980s was thus a time in which mental health services in Australia were exposed to intense public scrutiny. While the old system of segregated and custodial care was clearly in decline, and policymakers agreed on the need to establish a more balanced system that integrated hospital care with continuing care in community settings, public and professional support for the new directions seemed limited. It was against this backdrop of controversies and official inquiries into mental health services that the National Mental Health Strategy was developed and implemented.

The National Mental Health Strategy

Under Australia's federal system of government the role of the Commonwealth is largely restricted to co-ordinating the response to mental health issues nationally and to facilitating reform. Responsibility for the funding and delivery of mental health services mainly rests with the state and territory governments. The National Mental Health Strategy, which was a combined Commonwealth, state and territory initiative, was implemented in 1992. The main policy aims were to:

- promote the mental health of the Australian community and, where possible, prevent the development of mental health problems and mental disorders;
- reduce the impact of mental disorders on individuals, families and the community; and
- assure the rights of people with mental disorders.

(Australian Health Ministers, 1992a)

During the period 1992 to 1997 substantial gains were achieved in the range, quality, responsiveness and community orientation of mental health services. In particular, mental health services became a much more integrated component of mainstream health services. However, improvements were less than expected in a number of areas: access to services remained difficult in many regions, especially in rural and remote locations; primary care providers pointed to the continuing insularity of mental health services; the quality of services remained uneven within and across jurisdictions; and the extent of stigma and discrimination remained unabated for those with mental illness (Commonwealth Department of Health and Aged Care, 2000: 11). That indigenous Australians continue to experience much poorer health, including mental health, than the general population continues to be a major concern for both policymakers and health service providers (Australian Institute of Health and Welfare, 2000).

More recently priority has shifted to reforms in mental health promotion and prevention; to building partnerships in service reform; and to further enhancing service quality and effectiveness. Moreover, with formal recognition of the high level of unmet need for mental health care (Andrews and Henderson, 2000; Jablensky et al., 2000), the initial policy focus on the long-term mentally ill has been extended to take account of population health issues (Commonwealth Department of Health and Aged Care, 2000: 14).

Without doubt, the reforms have been most beneficial in increasing expenditure on mental health care and improving service mix. Funding for mental health services (not including disability support and housing) increased by 30% between 1992 and 1998. In the financial year 1997–1998 about 6% of overall health expenditure was allocated to mental health services (AU$2.24 billion). Within this overall increase in funding for mental health services, there was a significant expansion of community and general hospital services, while stand-alone psychiatric hospital services were reduced. In 1992–1993 only 29% of state mental health resources were allocated to services based in the community, and about half the total mental health expenditure of the states and territories was directed towards the provision of psychiatric beds in stand-alone hospitals. Between 1992 and 1998 spending by state and territory governments on community mental health services increased by 87%; at the same time a significant reduction occurred in the number of public sector psychiatric in-patient beds, from 45.5 beds per 100,000 in 1993 to 33.7 beds per 100,000 in 1998 (Whiteford et al., 2002). In the period 1991–1992 to 1997–1998 the number of public psychiatric hospitals reduced from 45 to 24, and the number of available beds in these facilities declined from 7,226 to 3,122 (Australian Institute of Health and Welfare, 2000: 267).

Unfortunately, the progress made in bringing increased resources and operational improvements to mental health services has not been matched in other key policy areas, such as assuring the human rights and citizenship entitlements of service users. While the various state and territory mental health acts have been improved, both in terms of human rights protection and consistency across jurisdictions, changing the letter of the legislation is no guarantee of enforcement in practice (Watchirs, 2000). There is little evidence that headway is being made in addressing such human rights concerns as: ignorance about the nature and prevalence of mental illness in the community; discrimination against people with a mental illness; misconceptions about the number of people with mental illness who are dangerous; and the belief that few people affected by mental illness ever recover (Human Rights and Equal Opportunity Commission, 1993). Despite a decade of reform under the National Mental Health Strategy, mental illness continues to be a 'deeply dehumanizing, culturally dispossessing and radically alienating' experience for many people (Johnstone, 2001: 200).

Within a policy context of balancing protection for the rights of people with mental illness with the 'need for treatment and the community's legitimate expectation to be protected from harm' (Whiteford et al., 2000: 413), much of the direction of reform continues to be shaped by the needs of specialist psychiatric services and the compulsory end of the treatment spectrum. Thus, while independent administrative mechanisms have been established to review treatment orders, to inspect in-patient services, or to investigate complaints, at a more general level the rehabilitation, housing and support services necessary for adjustment to life in the community remain seriously underdeveloped (Jablensky et al., 2000: 235).

Clearly, for many people with mental illness the reforms of the last decade have not brought social justice; all too frequently the experience of mental illness continues to be accompanied by the denial of entitlements that other citizens take for granted, including 'a sense of place in an intersubjective world, empathetic connection with reciprocating others, peace of mind, happiness [and] participatory citizenship' (Johnstone, 2001: 200). Among many service users, their families and mental health professionals there is an ongoing suspicion that 'the use of statements of civil liberties and consumer rights [is] little more than an empty political gesture' (Coffey, 1994: 35).

Citizenship and mental health reform

One way of assessing the extent of progress in achieving the aims of the National Mental Health Strategy is to ask whether those with mental illness are now better able to achieve the entitlements of citizenship. The concept of citizenship is usually understood as a combination of social rights and obligations that determines legal identity, access to scarce resources and social membership (Turner, 1990). Social commentators have identified a number of components of citizenship, including legal status (e.g. formal citizenship, rights and duties), social membership (e.g. access to institutions, services and resources), and civil ethics (e.g. sense of social responsibility, being a good neighbour) (Burke and Salvaris, 1997). Effective functioning in each of these domains indicates the extent of a person's social and civic well-being.

In liberal-democratic nations such as Australia, the notion of citizenship is often associated with expectations of self-sufficiency. If citizens have (civil, political, and social) rights, they also have obligations. Thus, while citizens enjoy a range of freedoms, they are also expected to be responsible for their own economic, social and emotional well-being. 'Good citizens' are expected to be financially secure, socially engaged and civic minded. While these civic virtues may be affected by any serious health problem (Turner, 1999), the impact of a mental disorder is likely to be especially disruptive.

Effective social and civil participation requires the building up of a complex set of life skills and knowledge over many years, ranging from the basic capacity for self-care through to communication skills, occupational skills, intellectual skills, human relationship skills and many others. Mental illness can seriously affect performance in each of these areas, resulting in a diminished sense of one's place in the community. And once these civil, social and political rights and responsibilities are eroded or lost through mental illness, they are not easily restored. Indeed, the distressing psychological, emotional and physical problems associated with mental illness are often compounded by severe restrictions in citizenship entitlements that result from prejudice associated with having a psychiatric diagnosis. These may include, but are by no means limited to, restrictions in access to insurance and superannuation schemes, ineligibility for membership in boards and tribunals, and exclusion from opportunities for participation in employment, education and training (Human Rights and Equal Opportunity

Commission, 1993). As Johnstone (2001: 201) has argued, the 'culturally normative prejudice' associated with mental illness can be as 'constraining and brutal' as the experience of political oppression.

The link between citizenship and mental health has clearly been recognized by policymakers in Australia (Australian Health Ministers, 1992a; 1992b). Developing strategies for service user representation, protection against discrimination and the adoption of safeguards and rights, such as those outlined in the United Nations *Principles for the Protection of Persons with Mental Illness* (United Nations General Assembly, 1992), have been key initiatives within the National Mental Health Strategy. As another policy document, the *Mental Health Statement of Rights and Responsibilities* asserts, it is important to ensure that the needs of the mentally ill 'for care, protection and rights to treatment and rehabilitation are satisfied. The diagnosis of mental health problems or mental disorder is not an excuse for inappropriately limiting their rights' (Australian Health Ministers, 1991: ix). As is the case with other citizens, people with mental illness are to be given the 'opportunity to live, work and participate in the community to the full extent of their capabilities without discrimination' (Australian Health Ministers, 1992a: 16). In demanding effective human rights protection and access to the full range of entitlements of citizenship, some Australian mental health activists have insisted that mental health reform be viewed as an issue of the 'democratization of human services provision' (Deakin Human Services Australia, 1999: 201).

It is important that policymakers, managers and providers of clinical services acknowledge that the injustices faced by the mentally ill and their families and other carers are not mere abstractions, but are a lived reality (Deakin Human Services, 1999). Such experiences are often characterized by intense loneliness, the lack of meaningful human connection, intimacy and shared identity, and an 'often unnoticed struggle to be heard' (Johnstone, 2001: 201). Nevertheless, it has been suggested that the attitudes and therapeutic mindsets of service providers often play a large part in why it is that treatments fall short of desired beneficial outcomes, and why many people who use mental health services continue to find this engagement unsatisfactory (Coffey, 1994; Deakin Human Services Australia, 1999). While service user involvement in all aspects of service planning, delivery and evaluation has been made a priority (Australian Health Ministers, 1992a), policymakers have complained that initiatives designed to achieve this outcome are not being taken up in the mental health workforce. Much greater emphasis needs to be given to increasing the responsiveness of the workforce to the concerns, outlooks and needs of service users. Accordingly, the challenge for the mental health professions is to move beyond traditional treatment approaches to find ways of helping those who experience severe mental illness to assert their rights as citizens:

People with mental illness are primarily citizens, with full citizenship and social rights ... Acceptance of this tenet means that the disciplines working in mental health are now obliged to meet not only the professionally defined *needs* of a person with mental illness but also to recognize inherent civil, political and social *rights*' (emphasis in original)

(Deakin Human Services Australia, 1999: 12)

Mental health consumerism

As has been noted above, the need to safeguard the human rights and citizenship entitlements of people with mental illness has become a central aspect of mental health policy in Australia. However, the form of 'citizenship' envisaged by policymakers has been heavily influenced by the introduction of market-style competition into the provision of health care and other public benefits and services in the past few decades (Davis, 1992; Grace, 1991; Hicks, 1995), a development which, it will be argued, has serious implications for the social justice aims of the mental health reforms. There has been an expectation that encouraging providers to compete for purchasers' business will lead to the more efficient provision of health care, because funding will be directed towards services and organizations that operate efficiently (Shackley and Ryan, 1994). While the efficiency imperative has been of central concern to policymakers and managers (Davis, 1992), the success of market-styled reforms depends, to some extent, on whether patients will, or even can, act as 'consumers'.

If the application of a consumer model to health care raises important questions, this is especially so in the case of mental health services. Indeed, the possible life experiences that may accompany severe mental illness are difficult to reconcile with a notion of 'consumer choice'. Such life experiences may range from non-treatment, homelessness and poverty at one end of the spectrum, to involuntary hospitalization, forced treatment and being subjected to legal orders at the other end. Moreover, the users of mental health services do not have the same access to clinical knowledge as health professionals (Pilgrim and Rogers, 1993: 166), and unlike most other categories of health service user, they are constantly at risk of having legally mandated restrictions placed on their personal liberty (and other civil rights). Even 'voluntary' patients may face significant problems – including the threat of being made an involuntary patient – in negotiating the formal and informal structures of the mental health care system (Centre for Health Law, Ethics and Policy, 1994: 13–17). Moreover, the onus for claiming the substantive rights set down in policy seems to fall on the vulnerable individuals concerned, as 'consumers' of mental health services (Watchirs, 2000: 3). Contrary to what might be expected given the designation 'health consumer', it is not at all clear that people with mental illness are in a position to assertively negotiate and transact 'business' with those who provide mental health services.

It is also important to note that those who use mental health services often seem reluctant to accept the official designation of 'consumer', preferring instead to see themselves as 'service users', 'recipients', or 'survivors' (Campbell, 1999). For many, developments such as advocacy, complaints procedures, or more liberal mental health legislation have not secured the power to choose. As Campbell (1999: 18) suggests, treating the mentally ill as if they were consumers risks 'missing the essential nature of their experience. A journey through a shopping mall and a journey through mental health services are simply worlds apart'.

However, the field is dominated by an ideology that focuses on the needs and concerns of consumers and carers as individuals. This perspective has dominated due to the widespread acceptance of liberal discourses about mental illness that stress the importance of concepts such as liberty, freedom and autonomy. Although these are concepts that must inform mental health policy and reform, it is important that they are not allowed to undermine a more community-oriented approach. Citizens, including mental health consumers and carers, are not isolated members of an atomized society. There are such things as a sense of community, common membership of linguistic groups, and common cultural heritage. It is important that the collective ethos that such conceptions of citizenship imply are not neglected in the development and implementation of mental health policy reforms.

Professional power and mental health care

It has been suggested above that those who provide mental health services to patients have been slow to embrace the human rights and citizenship principles that are so central to the National Mental Health Strategy. However, the resistance of some mental health professionals to this aspect of the policy framework is understandable if placed in historical context. The era of the asylum is still within the living memory of many persons currently working in and receiving care from mental health services and, as Cawte (1998: 16) has recently noted, the asylum system was one in which psychiatric professionals were expected to be both 'therapists' and 'gaolers'. Traditionally, patients with mental illness have been passive recipients of services controlled by professionals who decided what was 'best' (Barham, 1992: 64). Moreover, it has often been noted that the maintenance of social and psychological distance between professionals and those receiving their services has been a defining feature of professional dominance (Deakin Human Services Australia, 1999: 11). It can be all too easy for psychiatric personnel to disregard the opinions of the mentally ill as irrational, invalid, or even biased towards professional opinions (see for instance, Pridmore, 1990).

Nonetheless, with the rise of the consumer movement in the 1960s and 1970s, various groups began to challenge the prerogative of professionals to make treatment decisions *for* patients (Lupton, 1993: 147). By the 1990s policymakers were insisting that professionals work in partnership with those for whom they provide services. However, to date there is little evidence that the recent reforms have been successful in bridging the psychological 'distance' between professionals and those receiving their services. Indeed, the work of commentators such as Baron (1987), Barham (1992) and Coffey (1994) suggests that psychiatric personnel are unlikely to be wholly supportive of liberalizing policy changes, and that their responses may well range from unenthusiastic quiescence to open hostility and resistance. Moreover, professional acknowledgement for the differences in life-experience between people living in 'consensual reality' and those living with mental illness is rare (and perhaps grudging). While struggle can often be a feature of the experience of both groups, in the case of the former this struggle has an audience, a social and historical context, and a connection with others. In the case of those with mental illness, the struggle is often silent, unwitnessed, unconnected and without a history (Johnstone, 2001: 201). It is not surprising then, that many service users continue to insist that 'the most adverse attitudes to those with mental illness [come from] their treating staff, those who "gatekeep" the facilities and services dealing with mental illness' (Deakin Human Services Australia, 1999: 11).

There is also a strong perception among many staff that initiatives to promote patients' freedom of movement and expression through the liberalization of ward policies and practices, and the use of minimal sedation, have added to the workload and made the job much more complex. Moreover, the active promotion of patients' rights and the introduction of formal complaints mechanisms within mental health administrative procedures can also be experienced by staff as casting doubts on their professional integrity (Coffey, 1994: 34). The closer public scrutiny of what happens in psychiatric services and a more acutely ill clientele has increased the risks for staff, and made psychiatric work more demanding. Indeed, issues of security and risk management have become important concerns for many staff working in Australian mental health services in the last decade (Clinton and Hazelton, 2000a; 2000b; Hazelton, 1999).

There is also evidence that the policy-driven pressures and tensions running through mental health services have also amplified the intensely political nature of psychiatric work. While at the broadest level, medical/psychiatric thought and practice continue to provide the template for 'how things should be done' in mental health services, as with other health services, this is constantly open to challenge, resistance and modification

(Turner, 1987: 221–3; Wicks, 1995). Non-medical personnel are able to draw upon a range of tactics and strategies to hold medical authority in check: they may forge strategic alliances with other non-medical occupations; medical treatment orders can be gradually modified or only partially implemented; and medically preferred treatment approaches may even be openly challenged by non-medical personnel. Patients undoubtedly get caught up in inter-occupational conflicts between staff, and can be marginalized or even 'demonized', especially if there is disagreement over the management of patients considered 'difficult' and/or 'dangerous' (Hazelton, 1999).

Future prospects

Almost a decade after the implementation of the National Mental Health Strategy it is not clear that the life circumstances of mentally ill persons are changing for the better. While the old system of asylum care has been replaced by a comprehensive range of services located in both hospital and community settings, there is little evidence that people with mental illness are beginning to enjoy greater access to the full range of entitlements of citizenship. As Campbell (1999) has suggested, whether or not the rights and responsibilities of citizenship (and to this should be added protection of human rights) can be made available to mentally ill people depends on more than the shelter, support and occupational opportunity provided by formal health and community services; much also depends on the attitudes that operate within those services and inform public opinion.

It is also important to appreciate how longstanding – perhaps ancient – fears regarding the perceived association between insanity and criminality continue to find expression in occasional moral panics over the 'risks' and 'threats' posed by mentally ill people living 'unsupervised' in the community. As the recent Australian newspaper headlines provided in Table 3.1 indicate, 'madness', 'badness', 'risk' and 'crisis' feature heavily in the framing strategies by which the media present news related to mental health to the public. These stereotypical images can be understood as key elements of a well-established media discourse on mental health (Hazelton, 1997).

Campbell (1999: 24) has recently expressed concern that the limits of public tolerance for mentally ill people living in the community may already have been reached. This may well have been the case in the UK, where, as Morrall shows in Chapter One, public concern over homicides perpetrated by mentally ill offenders reached 'panic' levels in the 1990s. Elsewhere Morrall (2000) has described how public concern over unsupervised mentally ill persons living in the community has recently contributed to the emergence of post-liberal mental health policies and legislation in the UK.

Table 3.1 Selected Australian newspaper headlines related to mental health

Newspaper headline	Source
Killings linked to health crisis. Psychiatrist fears overcrowding at Graylands Hospital	*The West Australian* 8 February 1999
Mental block	*The Weekend Australian* 8–9 July 2000
Ombudsman inquiry into mental health crisis	*The Weekend Australian* 17–18 November 2001
Killer on day trips. Insane man unguarded	*The West Australian* 1 December 2001
The forgotten ones. Mental health is in crisis and sending the sick on to the streets	*The Australian* 29 April 2002

In general terms, post-liberalism can be understood as the incorporation of laws, policies and practices aimed at identifying, monitoring and excluding groups thought to pose a threat to public order, especially where there is an actual or potential threat of violence. The defining characteristic of 'post-liberal' control measures is that they are radically authoritarian, but operate within a democratic framework (Morrall 2000; Morrall and Hazelton, 2000). While the ideas and concerns that characterize the post-liberal turn in the UK do not appear to have influenced the formulation of mental health policy in Australia, there are signs that the trend is having an impact at the service level, especially in in-patient settings.

In one of the ironies of the mental health policy directions taken in Australia in the last decade, the emergence of a human rights agenda in psychiatric care has coincided with the tightening up of security practices in many health facilities. Driven to some extent by legitimate concerns over staff safety, 'service improvements' have included: the introduction of closed-circuit television monitoring in many in-patient wards; a return to the use of security windows in rooms, and fences to close off courtyards and thoroughfares; the building of seclusion rooms (now known as 'intensive care' or 'high dependency' units); and the requirement that staff wear electronic duress alarms on duty. At the same time, some hospitals have engaged private sector security guards, and there are cases of these guards being called to 'assist' in the management of disturbed patients in mental health wards and emergency departments. Developments such as these provide insights into the ways in which staff may 'manage' the policy directions set down in the National Mental Health Strategy. Instead of simply implementing initiatives set down by policymakers, these may be modified, ignored or undermined by those involved in the delivery of services. Indeed, it may well be that new forms of surveillance and new security practices are being developed as a kind of paradoxical response to the liberalizing reforms codified in the National Mental Health Strategy (Hazelton, 1999).

Perhaps the most important recent indication of ongoing human rights issues, in spite of the National Mental Health Strategy, is the well-publicized case of mental patients being manacled to beds in some hospitals in South Australia (*The Australian*, 16 November 2001). In March 2002, following the establishment of an inquiry to investigate the South Australian controversy, and the scheduling of inquiries into mental health services in several other states, a coalition of peak community and mental health organizations, including the Australian Council of Social Services, SANE Australia and the Australian and New Zealand College of Psychiatrists, expressed concern that the mental health system was in crisis and called for a national inquiry into services for people with mental illness.

After almost a decade of mental health reform in Australia it might be concluded that there are limits to what can be achieved in this area through formal policy initiatives. Johnstone (2001) has recently argued that protecting human rights and achieving citizenship entitlements for people with mental health problems and disorders requires subversion of the normalized culture of prejudice and discrimination historically associated with mental illness. It may well be that grass roots-level social criticism and political activism provide the best hope for achieving human rights and citizenship entitlements for people with mental illness. Rather than engaging in (bureaucratically) structured participation in health (Willis, 1995) as 'health consumers', there is the option of lobbying for better services and making other demands through local mental health pressure groups (Cullen and Whiteford, 2001: 26). Johnstone (2001: 207) is thinking in these terms when she suggests the need for a systematic programme to dislodge and reframe 'the deep-seated and normalized prejudice' that continues to confront the sufferers and survivors of mental illness.

Such a programme would need to be addressed to multiple audiences, including: the sufferers and survivors of mental illness who consciously identify as a socially excluded group; other sufferers and survivors of mental illness who do not identify as being socially excluded; other members of socially excluded groups; and members of dominant groups (Johnstone, 2001). Engaging in this kind of struggle would require that the representatives of any mental health movement develop skills in effective protest, including working alone and in groups, forming strategic alliances, publicizing mental health as a public issue, and working with the media (Thornton et al., 1997).

While the National Mental Health Strategy has undoubtedly brought significant gains in some areas, so far there is little evidence that the human rights and citizenship entitlements referred to in policy can be enforced in practice. While specialist mental health services have been improved throughout the country, insufficient attention has been given to rehabilitation, housing, employment, and community support – the very services necessary to support community adjustment. At the time of writing, the second five-year implementation plan is drawing to a close, and there has been no announcement about whether or not the National Mental Health Strategy will be extended for a further period of time. It is to be hoped that there will be continuing support for the policy directions of the last decade and that much greater emphasis will be given to improving access to the mainstream resources necessary to ensure that 'the onset of a severe mental illness need no longer be a barrier to ordinary human recognition and the entitlements of citizenship' (Barham, 1992: 1000).

Summary

Mental health has been identified as a National Health Priority Area in Australia relatively recently. In the last decade, in a series of sweeping reforms Australian mental health services changed from providing mainly institutional to mainly community-based care for people with mental problems and disorders. The reforms have been co-ordinated through a National Mental Health Strategy, and implemented through successive five-year plans. Nevertheless, despite significant improvements in expenditure and service mix, the transition from institutional to community treatment has not yet brought significant improvements to the lives of many people with severe mental illness. To date there is little evidence of progress in combating discrimination and safeguarding the human rights and citizenship entitlements of those with mental illness. It has been argued that health professionals are one group that displays adverse attitudes to the mentally ill. Moreover, the failure to provide adequate community services in such areas as rehabilitation, housing, employment and community support has increased the burden faced by the families of the mentally ill. The success of the National Mental Health Strategy should be measured against the extent to which those with mental illness are better able to access the full range of entitlements of citizenship.

Further reading

Deakin Human Services Australia (1999) Learning Together: Education and Training Partnerships in Mental Health Service. Final Report. Prepared by Deakin Human Services Australia with funding from the Commonwealth Department of Health and Aged Care under the National Mental Health Strategy. Canberra: Australian Government Publishing Service.

Jablensky A, McGrath J, Herrman H, Castle D, Gureje O, Evans M, Carr V, Morgan V, Korten A, Harvey C (2000) Psychotic disorders in urban areas: An overview of the study on low prevalence disorders. Australian and New Zealand Journal of Psychiatry, 34: 221–36.

Johnstone MJ (2001) Stigma, social justice and the rights of the mentally ill: Challenging the status quo. Australian and New Zealand Journal of Mental Health Nursing, 10 (4): 200–9.

Hazelton M, Clinton M (2001) Mental health consumers or citizens with mental health problems? In Henderson S, Petersen A (Eds.) Consuming Health: The Commodification of Health Care. London: Routledge. pp. 88–101.

References

Andrews G, Henderson S (2000) Unmet Need in Psychiatry. Problems, Resources, Responses. Cambridge: Cambridge University Press.

Australian Health Ministers (1991) Mental Health Statement of Rights and Responsibilities. Canberra: Australian Government Publishing Service.

Australian Health Ministers (1992a) National Mental Health Policy. Canberra: Australian Government Publishing Service.

Australian Health Ministers (1992b) National Mental Health Plan. Canberra: Australian Government Publishing Service.

Australian Institute of Health and Welfare (2000) Australia's Health 2000: The Seventh Biennial Health Report of the Australian Institute of Health and Welfare. Canberra: Australian Institute of Health and Welfare.

Barham P (1992) Closing the Asylum. The Mental Patient in Modern Society. London: Penguin Books.

Baron C (1987) Asylum to Anarchy. London: Free Association Books.

Burke T, Salvaris M (1997) Measuring civil society: Citizenship benchmarks and indicators. Geelong: Centre for Urban and Social Research (Deakin University), Benchmarking Citizenship, Citizenship in Australia Series, 1: 65–102.

Campbell P (1999) The consumer of mental health care. In Newell R, Gourney K (Eds.) Mental Health Nursing. An Evidence-Based Approach. Edinburgh: Churchill Livingstone. pp. 11–26.

Cawte J (1998) The Last of the Lunatics. Melbourne: Melbourne University Press.

Centre for Health Law, Ethics and Policy (1994) Model Mental Health Legislation. A Discussion Paper. Centre for Health Law, Ethics and Policy: The University of Newcastle, Australia.

Clinton M, Hazelton M (2000a) Scoping the Australian mental health nursing workforce. Australian and New Zealand Journal of Mental Health Nursing, 9 (2): 56–64.

Clinton M, Hazelton M (2000b) Scoping practice issues in the Australian mental health nursing workforce. Australian and New Zealand Journal of Mental Health Nursing, 9 (3): 100–9.

Coffey G (1994) Madness and postmodern civilization. Arena, April–May: 32–7.

Commonwealth Department of Health and Aged Care and Australian Institute of

Health and Welfare (1999) National Health Priority Areas Report: Mental Health 1998 – Summary. AIHW Cat. No. PHE 14. HEALTH and AIHW, Canberra.

Commonwealth Department of Health and Aged Care (2000) National Mental Health Report 2000: Sixth Annual Report. Changes in Australia's mental health services under the First National Mental Health Plan of the National Mental Health Strategy 1993–1998. Canberra: Australian Government Publishing Service.

Crichton A (1990) Slowly Taking Control? Sydney: Allen and Unwin.

Cullen M, Whiteford H (2001) The Interrelations of Social Capital with Health and Mental Health. Discussion paper. Canberra: Commonwealth Department of Health and Aged Care.

Davis A (1992) Economising health. In Rees S, Rodley G, Stillwell F (Eds.) Beyond the Market. Alternatives to Economic Rationalism. Leichhardt: Pluto Press.

Dax EC (1975) Australia and New Zealand. In Howells JG (Ed.) World History of Psychiatry. New York: Brunner Mazel. pp. 704–20.

Deakin Human Services Australia (1999) Learning Together: Education and Training Partnerships in Mental Health Service. Final Report. Prepared by Deakin Human Services Australia with funding from the Commonwealth Department of Health and Aged Care under the National Mental Health Strategy. Canberra: Australian Government Publishing Service.

Grace VM (1991) The marketing of empowerment and the construction of the health consumer: A critique of health promotion. International Journal of Health Sciences, 21 (2): 329–43.

Hazelton M (1997) Reporting mental health: A discourse analysis of mental health-related news in two Australian newspapers. Australian and New Zealand Journal of Mental Health Nursing, 6 (2): 73–89.

Hazelton M (1999) Psychiatric personnel, risk management and the new institutionalism. Nursing Inquiry, 6: 224–30.

Hicks N (1995) Economism, managerialism and health care. Annual Review of Social Science, 5: 39–60.

Human Rights and Equal Opportunity Commission (1993) Human Rights and Mental Illness. Report of the National Inquiry into the Human Rights of People with Mental Illness. Canberra: Australian Government Publishing Service.

Jablensky A, McGrath J, Herrman H, Castle D, Gureje O, Evans M, Carr V, Morgan V, Korten A, Harvey C (2000) Psychotic disorders in urban areas: An overview of the study on low prevalence disorders. Australian and New Zealand Journal of Psychiatry, 34: 221–36.

Johnstone MJ (2001) Stigma, social justice and the rights of the mentally ill: Challenging the status quo. Australian and New Zealand Journal of Mental Health Nursing, 10 (4): 200–9.

Lewis M (1988) Managing Madness: Psychiatry and Society in Australia 1788–1980. Australian Institute of Health. Canberra: Australian Government Publishing Service.

Lupton D (1993) Back to bedlam? Chelmsford and the press. Australian and New Zealand Journal of Psychiatry, 27: 140–8.

McDonald D (1983) Hospitals for the insane in the young colony. In Pearn J, O'Carrigan J (Eds.) Australia's Quest for Colonial Health. Some Influences on Early Health and Medicine in Australia. Brisbane: Department of Child Health, Royal Children's Hospital, Brisbane. pp. 183–90.

Morrall PA (2000) Madness and Murder. London: Whurr.

Morrall PA, Hazelton M (2000) Architecture signifying social control: The restoration of asylumdom in mental health care? Australian and New Zealand Journal of Mental Health Nursing, 9 (2): 89–96.

Pilgrim D, Rogers A (1993) A Sociology of Mental Health and Illness. Buckingham: Open University Press.

Pridmore S (1990) Mental health in the 1990s. Mental Health in Australia, 3 (1): 38–40.

Shackley P, Ryan M (1994) What is the role of the consumer in health care? Journal of Social Policy, 23 (4): 517–41.

Stoller A, Arscott KW (1955) Mental Health Facilities and the Needs of Australia. Canberra: Australian Government Printing Office.

Thornton P, Phelan L, McKeown B (1997) I Protest! Fighting for Your Rights. A Practical Guide. Annandale, New South Wales: Pluto Press.

Turner BS (1987) Medical Power and Social Knowledge. London: Sage.

Turner BS (1990) Outline of a theory of citizenship. Sociology, 24 (2): 189–217.

Turner BS (1999) Citizenship and health as a scarce resource. In Germov J (Ed.) Second Opinion. An Introduction to Health Sociology (revised edition). Melbourne: Oxford University Press. pp. 302–14.

United Nations General Assembly (1992) Principles for the Protection of Persons with Mental Illness and for the Improvement of Mental Health Care. New York: United Nations.

Watchirs H (2000) Application of Rights Analysis Instrument to Australian Mental Health Legislation. Report to the Australian Health Ministers' Advisory Council National Mental Health Working Group. Canberra: Commonwealth Department of Health and Aged Care.

Whiteford H, Thompson I, Casey D (2000) The Australian mental health system. International Journal of Law and Psychiatry, 23 (3–4): 403–17.

Whiteford H, Buckingham B, Manderscheid R (2002) Australia's National Mental Health Strategy. British Journal of Psychiatry, 180: 210–15.

Wicks D (1995) Nurses, doctors and discourses of healing. Australian and New Zealand Journal of Sociology, 31 (2): 122–39.

Willis K (1995) Imposed structures and contested meanings: Policies and politics of public participation. Australian Journal of Social Issues, 30: 211–27.

Chapter four

Italy: Radical reform of mental health policy and its consequences

Lorenzo Burti

Introduction

Recent Italian mental health policy has been deeply influenced by the radical reform of 1978 which, in turn, was uniquely conditioned by the experience of more than a decade-long exceptional deinstitutionalization movement. Thus, the understanding of present scenarios requires an adequate historical account, which makes up a considerable portion of this chapter. A lengthy portrait is given of the psychiatrist Franco Basaglia, the most symbolic, innovative and controversial personality of the reform movement.

Psychiatrists were the initiators of deinstitutionalization and the reform movement in Italy; they succeeded in steering other mental health workers, patients themselves, the labour unions, political parties and public opinion to support the cause of the liberation of mentally ill patients from asylums. At the same time mental health workers were struggling for their own emancipation as well, because until then they had been discriminated against by other health workers in terms of prestige, career and salary. This initial common struggle against the system may have paved the way for an alliance between mental health workers and users which still holds, and may account for the lack of harsh tones in consumer/survivor organizations, which often co-operate with the psychiatric system.

A concise description of the present situation of Italian psychiatry is given, with some reference to the context of the social and cultural situation of the country. Major studies providing relevant empirical data are then presented without any claim of completeness: basic reviews for further reading are quoted.

Historical background

Origins of Italian psychiatry

For centuries care of the mentally ill was provided by religious orders, according to the tradition of the Catholic church, in charitable initiatives for the poor and the disenfranchized. The modern psychiatric approach recognizes its founder in Vincenzo Chiarugi, who provided the Bonifacio Hospital in Florence with the kind of advanced and humanitarian regulations inspired by an Illuministic philosophy. For this Chiarugi is still remembered among the fathers of the modern institutional approach to the treatment of the insane. Italy became a state in 1861 but a national psychiatric law was issued only in 1904, when it was long needed after the exacerbation of problems of psychiatric care following the great institutionalization of the second half of the 14th century.

The 1904 Law No. 36: Provisions on Public and Private Mental Hospitals focused more on social control than treatment. Admission could only be involuntary, based on a diagnosis of dangerousness made by a physician and ordered by the police with a registration on the person's criminal records. An initial 30-day stay for evaluation would either lead to discharge or to permanent admission ordered by the court and implying the loss of civil rights. The law was soon criticized for its judicial aspects but nothing happened for decades, and during this time the number of psychiatric hospitals and their in-patient population increased dramatically. Figures peaked in 1963, with 98,544 psychiatric hospital beds, 91,868 in-patients on census day and a total of 34,199,000 hospital days in the year.

Deinstitutionalization

The treatment and care of the mentally ill in a humane and effective way, the prevention of mental illness, mental health promotion and, more generally, the improvement of the mental health status of all citizens entered the political domain only in the second half of the 20th century. This happened almost at the same time in several nations of the Western world in the late 1960s and early 1970s, propelled by student and worker protests. In Italy it was vigorously promoted by a group of radical psychiatrists led by Franco Basaglia, a young faculty member of the University of Padua School of Medicine, of existential-phenomenological orientation. He visited Maxwell Jones's therapeutic community in Scotland and was fascinated by the innovative approach. When he was assigned the directorship of the Psychiatric Hospital of Gorizia, a small city in northeastern Italy, with a group of dedicated colleagues sharing his ideas, he was shocked by the misery of the asylum and decided to reorganize the hospital according to the principles he had seen applied in the therapeutic community. However, soon, he and his colleagues realized that this would produce what seemed to them just a cosmetic change, because they believed the psychiatric hospital was the logical consequence of a more general process of social and political exclusion of the outcast. The group then decided to dismantle the psychiatric hospital which, in their eyes, appeared hopelessly anti-therapeutic. The ideas and accomplishments of this radical and still controversial group are accorded considerable space in this historical account because they left an impression on the Italian deinstitutionalization process by loading it with political meanings, and coupling an anti-psychiatric stance with a pragmatic approach. Other groups were active at the same time, but none was as innovative, successful or popular.

Actually the motto was one of 'dismantling the psychiatric hospital from within'. This set two important directions for the action to come and would eventually lead the nation to opt for a system *without* the psychiatric hospital. First, the group decided to dismantle the psychiatric hospital, rather than trying to improve it, in order to transform it into a therapeutic instrument. Basaglia and his group resolved early to cut the Gordian knot of the asylum, and this marked the most radical aspect of the reform: to do away with the psychiatric hospital *completely*. For decades to come, other nations would long debate the question of whether the psychiatric hospital could be improved and how. Some would even succeed in methodically emptying hospital after hospital, yet avoid ruling it out completely. Second, dismantling the hospital *from within* was Basaglia's idea, while other co-workers tried the other way around, i.e. to improve community services in order to drain the psychiatric hospital from outside. The former choice eventually proved to be the correct one: wherever alternative services were developed, in Italy and abroad, they tended to attract a different population. The most severely ill and marginal people remained in, or were re-hospitalized in, the psychiatric hospital.

Basaglia was, and still is, considered a member of the anti-psychiatry movement, but he always rejected such a definition. In reply to a direct question whether he and his group were anti-psychiatry, he stated: 'No, we are performing non-psychiatry' (Basaglia, 1968: 269). He was even critical of those on the most radical fringes of anti-psychiatry, especially Americans, fearing that their categorical defence of patients' individual freedom would possibly result in neglecting non-consenters.

In spite of popular anecdotes on supposed assertions that mental illness is simply a consequence of class divisions, Basaglia did not ultimately question its existence. He used the expression 'bracketing' applied to the term mental illness to stress his suspension of judgement on such an elusive construct that many still refrain from defining as a *disease*. He was concerned, instead, with the very tangible *consequences* of a psychiatric diagnosis applied to an individual from a low socio-economic class. When this individual is institutionalized, he loses all his rights: 'The patient, for the very fact of being admitted to an asylum, becomes, necessarily, a citizen without rights, entrusted to the power of doctors and nurses, who may do anything they wish with him, without any possibility of appeal' (Basaglia, 1968: 122). On the other hand, a well-to-do patient, with the same diagnosis, who is admitted to a private hospital, maintains most of his power and therefore has a reciprocal relationship, including a therapeutic one, with the doctor. Treatment is possible only within a reciprocal relationship, otherwise the proposed treatment is just another form of deceit and, ultimately, of violence. Therefore, the personnel of the institution should refuse to carry out their institutional mandate: they should 'deny' or 'negate' the institution, free the patients from anti-therapeutic captivity, and care for their real needs. The inscription 'Freedom is therapeutic' still greets visitors entering the hospital where Basaglia worked.

Therefore, with an unusually pragmatic attitude for an Italian, Basaglia and his co-workers set out to dismantle the psychiatric hospital from within, beginning with the most discriminating practices. Within a few years the hospital was completely transformed: all the wards and the hospital were opened to the free movement of patients and citizens and a programme of discharge was implemented. The model programme was later replicated in other cities. In Trieste Basaglia closed the psychiatric hospital and established a network of community-based services, demonstrating that it was possible to provide a comprehensive network of psychiatric services *without* the hospital. The achievements of this model programme had a tremendous impact on the liberal elites of mental health workers, intellectuals and students. The Association for Democratic Psychiatry was established, with a left political orientation. It managed to get the support of the labour unions and of the left-wing parties. This was a winning move, since the liberation of the mental patient was included in the agenda of social reforms brought forward especially by the Communist Party which, at the time, with more than 30% of votes, had reached an agreement with the Christian Democrats, the so-called 'Historical Compromise'. The movement's ideas became so influential that even the official Italian Psychiatric Association produced documents that rivalled the students' assembly proclamations in the use of radical jargon. In brief, there was a widespread agreement among mental health workers, lay people and public opinion at large on the urgent need for a change of the legislation dating back to 1904 and only marginally reviewed in 1968. In fact, the legislation supported an obsolete psychiatric system of services almost exclusively based on the psychiatric hospital, while ambulatory and especially community services were practically absent. Radical mental health workers were able to develop model programmes *in spite* of the archaic legislation and, especially, to bring the psychiatric problem into the political arena with the support of the Italian left. This definitely contributed to the creation of favourable conditions for legislative reform and inspired its formulation. Basaglia's ideas had such an impact on Law No. 180 (the reform law) that although he was never in the commission for the reform (he was only consulted) it is still nicknamed 'the Basaglia Law'. The connection with its radical (communist)[1] origins may explain why any discussion around the reform and its achievements, limits and alleged needs for change and integration remains as heated now as it was two decades ago.

The reform: Public Law No. 180 of 1978

The reform law was eventually written in a hurry and issued in May 1978, just in time to avoid a referendum promoted by the Radical party, which is small but very active in sponsoring liberal reforms. The government wanted to prevent an administrative void and a political setback.

The major characteristics of the reform were the following:

- The prohibition of building new psychiatric hospitals and the prohibition of using the existing ones for both the voluntary and involuntary hospitalization and rehospitalization of patients. As an exception, during a transition phase of two years, previously hospitalized patients could be admitted on a voluntary basis. After 1980, all admissions to psychiatric hospitals were prohibited. The status of all existing involuntary in-patients had to be reconsidered. However, the law incorporated no directive for their discharge. This prevented the risk of an abrupt discharge of large numbers of patients to the community, with all the related risks of abandonment, but left the whole initiative for their rehabilitation and reallocation to the goodwill of the personnel, practically allowing the indeterminate continuation of stay, albeit on a voluntary basis.
- The development of a comprehensive network of community mental health services responsible for the provision of all kinds of psychiatric interventions to the population of a given geographical area. Care in the community is defined as the preferred method of prevention, care and rehabilitation, while hospitalization is regarded as an exceptional intervention. All different components of the network must be integrated under an umbrella organization: the Department of Mental Health (DMH). Staff of psychiatric hospitals are to be transferred to the new services.
- Hospitalization, when necessary, has to take place in 15-bed general hospital units. The small number of beds is intended to avoid the settings becoming institution-like.

---

[1] Actually Basaglia never belonged to the Italian Communist party, the PCI, but certainly was close to the PCI and a representative of the Marxist intellectuals.

- Involutary hospitalization is allowed only when:
  - a psychiatric emergency occurs;
  - treatment is refused by the patient;
  - alternative community treatment is not effectively practicable.

Note that dangerousness is not mentioned as a requisite for commitment, because the aim is treatment of the patient, not public security. A number of legal procedures protect patient's rights: two independent medical evaluations are required; the provision is issued by a health officer and has to be ratified by a judge. The duration of involuntary admission is seven days, but extensions may be requested by the attending physician, who must advance justification for his decision to the judge. The patient him or herself or any other person may contest the decision in court. The patient's right to choose the physician and hospital must be granted as far as possible.

Within a few months Law 180 was incorporated in Law 833, which inaugurated the National Health Service (NHS). Thus the psychiatric reform became part of a major reform of the health system. The Italian NHS assures health care to all citizens through local administrations called USLs (*Unità Sanitarie Locali* [Local Health Units]) which are responsible for defined geographical areas of 50–200,000 inhabitants each.

Implementation of the reform

Laws 180 and 833 were just frameworks calling for national and regional implementation of legislation. Unfortunately, a national health plan was not passed until several years later and regions were quite uneven in the development of the new community-based services. The result was a patchy scenario with some areas well served, especially those where model programmes had been previously developed, in the north; however, the south of Italy long remained quite poor in services and resources. The pace of the reform was also affected by severe economic difficulties and the political instability that characterized Italy in the late 1970s after the assassination of Aldo Moro, the president of the Christian Democrats and principal creator of the Historical Compromise. All this helped to hamper the application of all social reforms passed in the decade, including Law 180. The inadequacy of alternative community services brought about opposition to Law 180, and several amendments were presented before parliament, although they did not get very far for the same economic reasons that hindered the implementation of the reform itself.

In spite of detractors' criticisms, a nationwide survey in 1984 revealed that a reasonable number of general hospital psychiatric units and community services existed and were accessible by about 80% of the Italian population in their own areas of residence. The number of in-patient care episodes was lower than before the reform, showing that blocking access to psychiatric hospitals did not precipitate a revolving door phenomenon in general hospital units. The number of admissions to private hospitals did not increase either; rather it remained stable or even decreased slightly. This demonstrated that a shift from hospital to ambulatory and community care in psychiatry was occurring. Residential facilities had been established as well but they were too few to meet the need for medium- to long-term residential care in a country with a hospital system designed for acute cases only: this was one of the major causes of discontent, especially among organizations representing families. In the meantime psychiatric hospital in-patients had decreased by one-half (from 60,000 to about 30,000) but quality of care and staff commitment had decreased as well.

Finally, a National Mental Health Plan was passed in 1994. It endorsed the policy of the reform and prescribed common standards and directions for financing the services. The DMH is responsible for planning, budgeting and running all psychiatric facilities and co-ordinating them with other health and social services. It comprises one or more psychiatric units with each unit serving a population of about 150,000. It has to be equipped with the following services:

1. A Community Mental Health Centre (CMHC), with out-patient and emergency care, family counselling, case management, social work, rehabilitation and vocational training.
2. One bed per 10,000 population in general hospital psychiatric wards (GHPW).
3. Semi-residential facilities with one bed per 10,000 population; residential facilities with at least one bed per 10,000 population (no more than 20 beds each); plus an extra bed per 10,000 population for the reallocation of former mental hospital in-patients.
4. Group homes where staffing should comprise at least one mental health worker per 1,500 population.

A new National Mental Health Plan was issued in 1998 with similar recommendations as to quotas, with a major emphasis on the integration of mental health services with other services and consumer organizations, plus quality assurance.

In the meantime, managed care policies started to influence mental health services more than other more profitable and less controversial medical specialties. Cuts in public funding gave momentum both to non-profit organizations in developing residential and semi-residential facilities and worker co-operatives, and to consumer self/mutual-help initiatives.

Eventually economics did away with the remaining psychiatric hospitals: the 1994 Financial Law successfully mandated the closure of all psychiatric hospitals by setting penalties for non-compliant regions.

Contemporary profile

Demographic and economic statistics

According to the National Institute of Statistics (Istat: http://www.istat.it) the present Italian population is currently 57,700,000, with an age structure comparable to that of other Western countries, i.e. with a growing representation of the elderly. Life expectancy at birth is 76 years for men and 82 years for women, and 17.7% of the population is 65 years and above. As to family structure, statistics report an average number of members per family of 2.7, a figure suggesting that the nuclear family is common. However, given reduced social mobility in comparison to other Western countries, various members of the extended family are geographically close, or even live in another apartment of the same building. In other words, the extended family is still a social reality in Italy, serving the purposes of contributing to child rearing, and caring for the elderly and disabled, including mental patients.

There has been an exponential increase of immigration from Africa, Eastern Europe and Asia in the last decade, which has introduced a sudden revolution within a demographically and socially dormant Italian society. There were 573,000 foreign residents in 1993, and 1,270,000 in 2000. The nation is experiencing unprecedented problems typical of multi-ethnic populations with episodes of racism and a growing chauvinistic inclination within some strata of society. Right-wing parties have taken advantage of the discontent for demographic and economic reasons. The public is increasingly dissatisfied with tax increases and drastic cuts in expenditures, which been adopted to reduce a previously reckless public debt and to comply with European recommendations. Thus, after years of unstable governments formed by coalitions of moderate and left-wing parties, the right has reached power, propelled by the popularity of Silvio Berlusconi.

For these reasons, in spite of the modest percentage of gross domestic product invested in health care (5.24%: 897 euros per capita per year), reforms to decrease expenses for welfare and health services are either in progress or planned, including proposals to repeal Law 180.

The Italian psychiatric services have been extensively described in the international literature (de Girolamo, 1989; Mosher and Burti, 1994; Tansella et al., 1998) and the present organization of psychiatric services has been recently reviewed by de Girolamo and Cozza (2000). A simple outline follows.

The closure of psychiatric hospitals

After almost two decades of stagnation, as an effect of the aforementioned 1994 financial law, between 1996 and 1998 26 psychiatric hospitals were closed and the number of patients dropped from 17,068 (on 31 December, 1996) to 7,704 (4,769 in public and 2,935 in private mental hospitals on 31 March, 1998). Eventually, all patients were accommodated in residential facilities developed *ad hoc*, either in hospital grounds or elsewhere.

Law 180 did not affect judicial mental hospitals, which many observers predicted would replace regular psychiatric hospitals in incarcerating severely ill and potentially dangerous mental patients. This did not happen: actually the number of in-patients in judicial mental hospitals has been steadily declining over the years (De Salvia and Barbato, 1993).

Community mental health centres (CMHCs)

A total of 695 CMHCs are reported as being operative in the country: 1.81 per 150,000 population. They are the headquarters of community psychiatry teams. At the beginning of the reform their distribution was patchy, and their organization and resources meant they operated as small clinics open a few hours a day in the majority of cases (although a few were multi-service centres with overnight beds and 24-hour emergency care) (Bollini and Mollica, 1989). At present, they are generally open 12 hours a day, 5–6 days a week, and offer the following interventions: evaluation, individual treatment planning, ambulatory care, home care, liaison with general practice, consultation, hospital (public and private) gate-keeping, and quality assurance. The staffing comprises multidisciplinary teams that include psychiatrists, psychologists, social workers, psychiatric nurses and other various paramedical staff including counsellors, teachers and occupational therapists. They were assigned, by the reform, the major responsibility of care to all psychiatric patients in their catchment area with one-year reported prevalence varying between 0.8 and 4.4 per 1,000 population according to different psychiatric registers (Veltro et al., 1993). Existing data also show that CMHCs are capable of serving, in the community, severely ill and socially deprived patients, mostly with a diagnosis of psychosis and repeated admissions (Marino et al., 1996; Mattioni et al., 1999). When outcome is considered in relation to the comprehensiveness of care and style of intervention, patients treated in comprehensive community services show better status at follow-up (Kemali and Maj, 1988). A prospective study of patients with functional psychoses in 76 out-patient centres showed that a substantial proportion had a favourable outcome (Terzian et al., 1997). In a study on satisfaction, patients and relatives receiving comprehensive community care expressed similar expectations and were mostly satisfied

(Ruggeri, 1996). While results of individual studies cannot be generalized, there seems to be a consistency in findings: where well-organized and comprehensive mental health services exist, community care is feasible and provides good outcomes, and users are satisfied. The style of intervention is mixed: medical, with a widespread use of medication; and psychosocial, with a careful use of welfare benefits supporting treatment interventions. Foreign observers are sometimes puzzled because they may misinterpret a friendly or even casual attitude of the staff toward the patients for a lack of professionalism. According to Lovell (1986) this is actually a sophisticated psychosocial, non-medical form of professional approach.

In-patient care

In-patient care is provided by 10,083 acute psychiatric beds (4,084 in general hospital psychiatric units [7 per 100,000 population, a figure close to the recommended standard of 10 per 100,000]; 404 in university departments; 5,595 in private hospitals) with an overall rate of 17 per 100,000 population. General hospital psychiatric units have to provide acute care for both voluntary and involuntary admissions. Admissions to general hospital psychiatric units are declining, with 278 per 100,000 population in 1987 and 222 in 1994, while those to private hospitals have remained stable, with 155 in 1975 and 140 in 1994. Notably, compulsory admissions decreased substantially (57 per 100,000 population [50% of all admissions in 1977] to 24 in 1984 [12% of all admissions]). About 60% of admissions carry a diagnosis of psychosis, thus confirming that hospitalization is regarded as an intervention for severe cases. The average length of stay varies between one and three weeks (Istat, 2000).

Day care

In the case of day care, 257 day hospitals (0.67 per 150,000 population) and 481 day centres (1.26 per 150,000 population) are reported. Both cover the need for semi-residential facilities: the former provide day evaluation and treatment and may be located in a hospital or at a CMHC; the latter are community-based and offer psychosocial treatment, and social and vocational rehabilitation. A considerable number of day care and vocational rehabilitation centres are run by private, non-profit co-operatives in a similar way to residential facilities (see below).

Staffing and training

The staffing of public services comprises 8.8 psychiatrists per 100,000 population, 3.0 psychologists, and 26.8 nurses. Since the reforms have been in place for some time most personnel previously transferred from psychiatric hospitals have now retired and only a few remain. Residual senior staff have developed experience in community care, and transfer their skills to their less experienced colleagues. Thus the most important phase of training takes place in the field. Education to prepare students for community work has improved: about half the Italian university psychiatric departments are more or less involved with community psychiatry and are therefore able to teach specific skills. In addition, new professional careers in the field of psychiatric rehabilitation and education of the disabled, and corresponding curricula, have recently been developed. Those currently graduating in these new careers have a far better training in community care and rehabilitation than their colleagues of the past.

Residential facilities

A recent survey identified more than 1,300 facilities with various levels of direct staff supervision, totalling about 17,000 beds (3 beds per 10,000 population). They are directly run either by the public system or by private, non-profit organizations under contract to the Department of Mental Health after satisfying criteria for accreditation.

Usually the residential facilities are family-like, but some are larger and more institutional. They generally offer rehabilitation in personal and social skills and achieve some success in preparing clients for more independent living arrangements (group homes, living alone or with family). These facilities represent the fastest growing segment of the system in the last decade, for many reasons. In the first place, there was a relative accumulation of patients in need of medium- to long-term residential accommodation, since the country does not have a hospital system for them; second, increased family burden was one of the major complaints after the reform; third, the void provided a market for the previously mentioned non-profit organizations, usually co-operatives. Some of them were already offering care for the disabled, but many more were established because of the expansion in the market. They are now organized at a national level and have their own system of training and peer review for quality assurance. A possible unwanted effect of this extensive participation of the private sector in residential care and rehabilitation is that the public system may eventually allocate rehabilitation to the private sector wholesale. In such a scenario, the public system might limit itself to biological treatment and hospital care with an eventual cultural impoverishment.

Worker co-operatives

Basaglia exploited the Italian model of co-operatives to provide real job positions to former psychiatric hospital patients. His ideas were expanded and there are now more than 400 co-operatives employing approximately 4,000 mentally ill patients. These succeed in competing commercially with normal companies thanks to incentives provided by advanced legislation. Law 381 of 1991 and subsequent legislation offers tax exemptions and direct contracting with public administrations to worker co-operatives employing at least one-third of handicapped employees.

Carer and patient groups

Family organizations were particularly vigorous in expressing dissatisfaction for the delayed development of community services in the early years after the passing of the reform law. They complained about carrying most of the burden of community care for mental patients with the respite of only brief admissions to the general hospital units. Especially critical was the shortage of day and alternative residential care. Some family organizations lobbied conservative mental health workers for a return to the old system and supported proposals to repeal the reform. However, some family organizations supported the reform and simply called for its full implementation.

According to the National Mental Health Plan, family organizations are regularly consulted when regulations are decided at national and regional levels, and should be invited to sit on DMH advisory boards, but this is not a diffuse practice. Since 1993 a number of family organizations gathered to form the National Union of the Associations for Mental Health (UNASAM), which is part of the national and international network of non-governmental organizations. The (ex-user self-help movement is rapidly expanding in Italy. Unlike the user/survivor organizations of other countries, which often express severe dissatisfaction with psychiatric services, Italian organizations generally collaborate with psychiatric services, possibly because of the user-friendly attitude of the Italian system.

Studies on burden and quality of life found that families reported difficulties including negative changes in family life, fatigue, and reduced family income (Gallio et al., 1991). A high level of burden was found among carers, including poor social relationships with others, depression and deteriorating physical health (Veltro et al., 1993). A cross-cultural study compared the support provided by carers, patients and families from Bologna (Italy) and Boulder (Colorado, USA) (Warner et al., 1998). In Bologna 74% of patients lived with their families, compared to 17% in Boulder. A better quality of life reported by Italian patients therefore seems to be an effect of the quality and quantity of family support received.

Recent policy initiatives

Four proposals have recently been submitted to parliament, all sharing a rebuttal of existing legislation and a call for the establishment of medium-to long-term *hospital* care (with institutions of up to 50 beds each) and more permissive norms for speedy involuntary admissions. Two are updated versions of previous proposals that were unsuccessful and which have now been re-submitted in the hope of taking advantage of a more conservative political leadership. The four proposals were eventually merged into one. The basis of the proposal results from popular complaints typically voiced by family organizations about the most controversial aspect of Law 180, i.e. the lack of hospital wards for medium- to long-term-stay patients and the consequent adverse effects of early discharge from overcrowded wards with a rapid turnover. This tends to occur where community care is inadequate: general hospital wards are overloaded by increased admissions and a lack of aftercare. In fact, since there is no set time-limit to the length of stay in general hospital psychiatric wards, in the case of severe behavioural problems, with a lack of alternative accommodation, patients may remain hospitalized for months or even years. The only limiting factor is the small number of beds. Thus hospitals rely on community services either to limit the number of admissions by caring for severe cases in the community, or for finding a place for them in one of the (many) home-like residential alternatives.

Discontent with delayed involuntary commitments has to do, again, with inefficient community services. Poor follow-up and community monitoring of chronic cases living in the community leads to a more frequent need for involuntary commitment. Effective community teams, instead, effectively monitor the course of illness and maintain a therapeutic alliance with their patients, thus reducing the incidence of relapse and the need for involuntary commitment. In brief, the community team is the critical component of the Italian system: where it does not operate properly, problems arise. Controversy is raging: supporters of the proposals state that the present situation is unbearable, while supporters of Law 180 insist that these proposals would practically cancel a quarter of a century of advances in community mental health care and bring Italy back to the use of asylum-like institutions. At the end of 2002 the unified proposal of reform came to a halt. This was the consequence of a growing, diffuse criticism expressed by professionals and lay people, some political disagreement even within the governmental coalition and, last but not least, the Italian economic recession. As has occurred in the past (see above), there are no funds to establish all the institutions that the reformers advocate.

Experiences

Giovanni, a former state hospital inmate and a patient of the South Verona Community Mental Health Services, said to a WHO inspector visiting the services: 'I was in the hospital for 12 years, and didn't like it. I prefer by far to live in my apartment and wish to express my appreciation to the workers for their respect and support. Let me recommend that action be taken internationally to develop community services instead of psychiatric hospitals. Workers and patients should be educated accordingly.' The WHO inspector was amazed: Giovanni ordinarily spoke only of his delusion of being a descendant of Julius Caesar; he had never spoken a complete sentence before.

Marisa, a veteran of psychiatric systems across the Atlantic (a Verona native who had married a US soldier), reported her experiences: 'Well, doctor, the state hospital in Tallahassee, Florida, was not so bad. They would let me go to town freely and even found me a paid job as a waitress.' When the author looked disheartened, Marisa continued: 'I was kidding, you are all okay, but tell Luciana (the social worker who administers Marisa's meagre pension and opposes her uncontrolled spending habits) to give my money back!'

Giuliana, a long-time member of a residential alternative (who used to live in her car for weeks before being brought to the emergency room in a coma for untreated diabetes) said: 'I would rather have my own apartment but here it is for free!' Eventually she was assigned a low-priced apartment from the municipality and lives on her own, but visits her former comrades at the residence almost daily.

Nicoletta, a guest of another hostel, says, 'No, I do not like the hospital. I like this place much better. We are all friends here. I do not like staff wearing a white coat.'

The sister of Alberto, a young patient with a recent diagnosis of schizophrenia, in a dramatic session of a relatives' group shouts, 'You doctors aren't doing any good to my brother, you just drug him. He should work, but he doesn't even have the energy to get up and look for a job! What kind of rubbish are you giving him?' Alberto's mother nods, in silence, evidently furious.

'I know that my daughter won't ever be well,' intervenes the mother of Laura, a woman with a resilient form of schizophrenia, a typical non-responder, 'you must learn to get along with this; some things can change, others cannot, no matter what you do. You simply have to take them as they are. These meetings have helped me to make sense and put together all the ideas I have developed on my own over the years. Thank you doctor.'

'In the group [a self-help group], patients are really different. They aren't sick any more,' says a young resident during his visit to the most recent initiative – a collaborative project between psychiatric services, a non-profit worker co-operative and a consumer self-help association. 'They are people. I don't hear about symptoms; they are competently speaking about work to be done, income, commercial projects – all normal things!'

Summary and conclusions

There are two opposite attitudes in writing concluding remarks on a controversial experience such as the Italian one: non-aligned and opinionated. The first is by far the most widely used by Italian authors when publishing in the international literature. Impartiality better resembles the objectivity commanded by modern empirical science. However, whether the basic dilemma in choosing between alternative psychiatric systems may be disentangled either on scientific or political grounds, is open to discussion.

The Italian reform was passed for cultural and political reasons in a specific historical context, but reflects the widely accepted principles of community psychiatry: it simply stretched such principles enough to include the closure of all psychiatric hospitals. The development of necessary alternative services and the accumulation of experience by community teams required time. Presently Italy has the most comprehensive and diffuse disseminated network of community psychiatric services than any other country in the world. Persistent differences in the distribution of resources call for improvement but, in the opinion of a vast number of workers and users, do not imply the repeal of existing legislation. In those many areas where the reform has been applied, empirical evidence proves the effectiveness of community services in meeting all psychiatric needs, including those of the severely mentally ill and their families.

References

Basaglia F (Ed.) (1968) L'istituzione Negata. Torino: Einaudi.

Bollini P, Mollica RF (1989) Surviving without the asylum: An overview of the studies on the Italian reform movement. Journal of Nervous and Mental Disease, 177: 607–15.

de Girolamo G (1989) Italian psychiatry and reform law: A review of the international literature. International Journal of Social Psychiatry, 35: 21–37.

de Girolamo G, Cozza M (2000) The Italian psychiatric reform. A 20-year perspective. International Journal of Law and Psychiatry, 23: 197–214.

De Salvia D, Barbato A (1993) Recent trends in mental health services in Italy: An analysis of national and local data. Canadian Journal of Psychiatry, 38: 195–202.

Gallio G, Morosini PL, Veltro F (1991) Malattia mentale e carico famigliare: Analisi di un campione di famiglie di utenti dei servizi di salute mentale di Trieste. Paper presented at the 38th National Congress of the Italian Psychiatric Association, 1991.

Istat (2000) Statistiche della sanità: Anno 1997. Rome: Istituto Nazionale di Statistica.

Kemali D, Maj M (Eds.) (1988). Attuazione della legge di riforma e valutazione dei servizi psichiatrici in Italia. Rivista Sperimentale di Freniatria, 112 (Suppl. 3): 597–682.

Lovell AM (1986) The paradoxes of reform: Re-evaluating Italy's mental health law of 1978. Hospital and Community Psychiatry, 37: 802–8.

Marino S, Frattura L, De Luca LF, De Francesco M, Olivieri M, Saraceno B (1996) The provision of psychiatric care in Southern Italy. Results from the Psychiatry in Southern Italy's Services (de PISIS) survey. International Journal of Social Psychiatry, 42: 181–92.

Mattioni T, Di Lallo D, Roberti R, Miceli M, Stefani M, Maci C, Peducci CA (1999) Determinants of psychiatric inpatient admissions to general hospital psychiatric wards: An epidemiological study in a region of central Italy. Social Psychiatry and Psychiatric Epidemiology, 34: 425–31.

Mosher LR, Burti L (1994) Community Mental Health. New York: Norton.

Ruggeri M (1996) Users' satisfaction with psychiatric services. In Thornicroft G, Tansella M (Eds.) Mental Health Outcome Measures. Berlin: Springer-Verlag. pp. 27–52.

Tansella M, Amaddeo F, Burti L, Garzotto N, Ruggeri M (1998) Community-based mental health care in Verona, Italy. In Goldberg D, Thornicroft G (Eds.) Mental Health in our Future Cities, Maudsley Monographs No. 42. London: Psychology Press. pp. 239–62.

Terzian E, Sternai E, Barbato A, Tognoni G, Saraceno B (1997) Epidemiology of psychiatric care of patients with severe mental disorders in Italy. Rationale and design of a prospective study, and characteristics of the cohort. Social Psychiatry and Psychiatric Epidemiology, 32: 298–302.

Veltro F, Magliano L, Lobrace S, Morosini PL (1993) Severely and persistently mentally ill patients in Italy: An overview of epidemiological and psychosocial findings. International Journal of Social Psychiatry, 39: 285–302.

Warner R, de Girolamo G, Belelli G, Bologna C, Fioritti A, Rosini G (1998) Quality of life and psychopathology in Boulder, Colorado, and Bologna, Italy. Schizophrenia Bulletin, 24: 559–68.

CHAPTER FIVE

Egypt: 5000 years of science and care for mental patients

AHMED OKASHA

Introduction

The Egyptian constitution states that basic services such as health and education should be made accessible to all citizens, free of charge and with no discrimination on the basis of gender, religion or race. As such the constitution sets two basic conditions for the provision of health care, inclusive of mental health care – namely, accessibility and non-discrimination, two basic elements of human rights. However, documents and statements are not enough to guarantee the implementation of their provisions. Economic policies, social change and, foremost, social attitude towards a phenomenon such as mental illness constitute major factors that may hinder or facilitate the implementation of those provisions. This chapter reviews the historical developments of the cultural and professional attitude towards the mentally ill, the current situation regarding availability and quality of mental health care services, and the future expectations based on the most recent mental health policy adopted by the Ministry of Health for the promotion of mental health in Egypt.

Historical background

During Pharaonic times, mental illness was not known as such, as there was no separation between soma and psyche. Actually, mental disorders were described as symptoms of diseases of the heart and uterus, as stated in Eber's and Kahoun's papyri. In spite of the mystical culture, mental disorders were attributed and treated on a somatic basis. Consequently there was no stigma associated with mental illness, as mental disorders were considered to be physical in nature and were treated in the same site (Okasha, 1999a).

In the Islamic era the approach to mental illness was based on two main sources:

1. The Holy Text (the Koran): The most common word used to refer to the mad person, i.e. insane or psychotic, in the Koran is *majnoon*. This is mentioned five times in the Koran to ascribe how prophets were perceived.
2. Common convictions at the popular level: The same word is used by the masses to describe the perceived eccentricity of all prophets when they attempt to guide their people to enlightenment. It is sometimes coupled with being a magician or a teacher. In a sense, there seems to be a positive connotation to madness that would flatter the anti-psychiatry concept of madness, which flourished in the mid-1960s (Shaalan, personal communication, 1989).

The word *majnoon* is originally derived from the word *jinn* (the word *jinn* in Arabic has a common origin with overlapping words with different connotations and can refer to a shelter, screen, shield, paradise, embryo and madness). The current Islamic concept that the insane person is possessed by a *jinn* should not be confused with the concept of the Middle Ages. In Islam, the *jinn* is not necessarily a demon, i.e. an evil spirit. It is a supernatural spirit, lower than the angels, that has the power of assuming human and animal forms, and can be either good or bad. Some *jinn* are believers who listen to the Koran and help human fairness. Moreover, Islam is not devoted to human beings but also to the spiritual world at large. In the Koran, almost always, the *jinn* and the human being are mentioned together. This has altered the concept and the management of the insane. Insane people may be perceived as being possessed but the possession may be by a good or a bad spirit. Consequently there was no place to generalize punishment or to give condemnation unconditionally.

Apart from the concept of the insane being possessed, there is another positive concept where the insane person is taken as the one who dares to be innovative, original and creative or attempts to find alternatives to a static and stagnant mode of living. It is also to be found in various attitudes towards certain mystics such as in Sufism, where the expansion of self and consciousness has been taken as a rationale to label some of the Sufis as psychotic. The autobiographies of some Sufis reveal the occurrence of psychotic symptoms and many mental sufferings in their paths to self-salvation (Rakhawy, personal communication, 1989).

The third concept of mental illness is the consequence of the disharmony or constriction of consciousness, which 'non-believers' are susceptible to. It is related to the denaturing of the basic psychic structure and disruption of a harmonious existence by egoism, detachment or alienation, partly presented by the loss of integrative insight. This can be more easily understood if we became acquainted with the essence of Islam as an existential mode of living, behaving and relating to nature, and the basic belief in the beyond – not necessarily supernatural.

The prevailing concept of mental illness at a particular stage in the Islamic world had always depended on the dominance of development or deterioration of genuine Islamic issues. For instance, during deterioration, the negative concepts of the insane as being possessed by evil spirits dominate, whereas during periods of enlightenment and creative epochs, the disharmony concept dominates, and so forth. The prevailing interpretation affected the attitude of the society as well as the profession and the quality of service provided for the mentally ill.

Islam also identified the unity of body and psyche. The psyche is mentioned 185 times in the Koran as a broad reference to human existence, meaning at different times body, behaviour, affect, and/or conduct, that is, total psychosomatic unity.

The teaching of the great clinician Rhazes had a profound influence on Arab as well as European medicine. The two most important books of Rhazes are *El Mansuri* and *Al-Hawi*. The first consists of 10 chapters, including the definition and nature of temperaments and comprehensive guides to physiognomy. *Al-Hawi* is the greatest medical encyclopaedia produced by a Moslem physician. It was translated into Latin in 1279 and published in 1486. It is the first clinical book presenting the complaints, signs, differential diagnosis and the effective treatment of illness. One hundred years later, Avicenna's monumental educational and scientific book, *El-Canoon* was published and this contained a better classification.

The first Islamic hospital appears to have been established in the early 9th century in Baghdad and to have been modelled on the East Christian institutions, which seem to have been mainly monastic infirmaries.

Among the hospitals that appeared throughout the Islamic world, perhaps the most famous was the one created in Cairo by the Egyptian Sultan al-Mansour Kalaoon in 683/1284. It was a richly endowed monumental structure that attracted the interest of foreign visitors to Cairo until the 19th century. The hospital, in the centre of Cairo, was formerly a Fatimid palace, which explains its plan and ornate decoration. It formed, moreover, part of a complex that included the mausoleum of the Sultan, a mosque, a school and baths. This structure alone indicates the integration of mental health care into other services, reflecting an attitude of acceptance and empathy.

The Egyptian historian al-Maqrizi, who wrote in the early 15th century, gives a full description of the Bimristan al-Mansuri, sometimes called the Bimristan of Kalaoon or simply Dar Ash-Shifa [house of healing]. Al-Maqrizi says that the reason for the Sultan's foundation was that in 675/1276, when he was a prince fighting the Byzantine, he was attacked by severe colic in Damascus and the doctors treated him with medicines brought from the Nur ad-Din hospital. Al-Mansur recovered and went to inspect the hospital; he admired it and vowed that, if God made him King, he would build such a hospital. Soon after, in 678/1279, he became Sultan of Egypt and began the construction of his hospital (Dols, 1992).

The 14th century Kalaoon Hospital in Cairo had departments for surgery, ophthalmology, and medical and mental illnesses. Contributions by the wealthy of Cairo allowed a high standard of medical care and provided for patients during convalescence until they were gainfully occupied. Two features were remarkable: the care of mental patients in a general hospital, and the involvement of the community in their welfare – an approach that predated modern trends by six centuries (Baashar, 1975). Care for the mentally ill was the responsibility of the community at large, securing quality and access.

According to al-Maqrizi:

When the building was finished, al-Malik al-Mansour endowed it with the revenue from several properties in Cairo and other places that amounted to about 1,000,000 dirhams a year. He provided funds for the hospital, the mausoleum, the school and an orphanage. Afterwards, the Sultan secured the drugs, doctors, and everything that was necessary for the sick in the hospital. He appointed attendants of both sexes to serve the sick, and set their wages. He provided beds with mattresses and everything that was needed by the sick. He set apart a special place for each kind of illness. Thus, parts of the hospital were designated for those with fevers and similar illnesses. He assigned a hall for an oculist, a hall for a surgeon, a hall for those with diarrhoea, a hall for women, and a place for those who had a cold temperament (i.e. the insane). The latter were divided into two sections, one for men and the other for women. He had running water installed in all parts of the hospital and areas were designated for the kitchen, medications, potions, and preparing electuaries, collyria, eye powders, and similar things, as well as places for storing these products and for distributing drugs and drinks. He also made a place in the hospital for the head of the physicians for the reading of medical texts. The number of admissions to the hospital was not fixed; all had access to it, without distinction between rich and poor. Also, the duration of treatment was unlimited, and even at home the sick received all the medications that they needed.

(Dols, 1992)

Recommended treatment for the mentally disturbed usually included baths, fomentation (particularly to the head), compresses, bandaging, and massage with various oils. Blood-letting, cupping, and cautery were also widely used. A familiar term for an antidepressant in the medieval period was *mufarrih an-nafs* [gladdening of the spirit], which was expected to relieve the patient's sadness. According to Ibn Abi Usaybia's account, al-Tamimi, a 10th century doctor, had concocted a drug called 'the key to joy from every sorrow and the gladdening of the spirit' [*miftah as-surur min kull al-humum wa mufarrih an-nafs*]. The production of such drugs had had a long tradition since antiquity. Incidentally, because one of the ingredients was crushed rubies, *mufarrih* was a common subject of oriental love poetry: the lovesick hoped for the healing of his passion by the ruby lips of his beloved (Burgel, 1972).

According to Ibn Sina'a the purpose of the diets, baths and medications was to increase the moisture of the body in opposition to the presumed drying effect of the black or burnt bile. Cold and moist foods were also advised as a corrective to burnt yellow bile, the major cause of mania; whey, particularly, was highly recommended on the authority of Galen. The purpose of blood-letting and purgatives was to evacuate the damaging black bile. Drugs were obviously intended to calm the excited, stimulate the apathetic and comfort the depressed (Dols, 1992).

The beneficial effects of music for healing had been widely acknowledged since antiquity. Musical performances were often given at the Mansuri Hospital in Cairo; one of the designated expenditures was for troops of musicians to come each day and entertain the patients. During the Ottoman period, the older hospitals continued to employ music, and the Turkish ones were remarkable for continuing the practice.

It appears that other forms of diversion were also used in the hospital, such as dancing, theatrical performance, and recitation. Patients suffering from insomnia were placed in a separate hall; they listened to harmonious music, and skilled storytellers recited their tales to them. When the patients began to recover their sanity, they were isolated from the others, and dancing and various sorts of comedies were staged for their benefit. When they left the hospital, the patients were given five gold pieces, so that they were not obliged immediately to return to work.

Similarly, care was taken about the quality of the air, which was scented with herbs; immense fans called *pankas* were used to circulate the air, and the floors were covered with branches of henna, pomegranate, mastic and fragrant vines. The famous balsam from Heliopolis was reserved for the hospital for the medication of the patients.

Nevertheless, the basic responsibility for the insane lay with the family. The Koran and Islamic law strongly reinforced this ancient duty. The Koran states: 'Do not give to the incompetent their property that God has assigned to you to manage; provide for them and clothe them out of it; and speak to them honourable words.'

In the early 19th century, during the French occupation of Egypt, the director of medical services in the Egyptian armed forces, a French physician named Claude, approached the Egyptian ruler regarding the appalling state of mental patients in Cairo. At that time all medical hospitals were under military control, so mental patients in Cairo were transferred to a military hospital in the middle of the city (al-Azbakia). After a few years, they were transferred to a nearby independent building in Bab el-Louk. In 1880, a fire destroyed one of the Royal palaces except for a two-storey building. This was painted yellow and became the first mental hospital in Cairo in 1883. It was called the Yellow Palace and at that time it was situated in Abbassia, a remote desert suburb of Cairo. In 1912 another state mental hospital was built in Khanka, several kilometres to the north of Cairo. It occupied about 300 acres and included a large plantation (Okasha, 1993).

Since their establishment the Abbassia (100 years ago) and Khanka (80 years ago) mental hospitals had British directors until the early 1930s. A report dating back to 1920 about the psychiatric services in Egypt was signed by John Warnock and HW Dudgeon, the directors of Abbassia and Khanka mental hospitals, respectively. The report includes a list of the prevalent psychiatric diagnoses at that time; in decreasing frequency, these were: adolescent insanity, pellagra, alcohol, syphilis, congenital abnormalities, old age, hashish and epilepsy. Other diagnoses were mentioned to a lesser extent: fevers, cocaine and the puerperium as well as mental stresses such as grief and loss. Yet the majority of cases were listed as of unknown aetiology (Warnock and Dudgeon, 1920). In 1920, Egypt had 12 psychiatric beds for every 100,000 population. Beginning in 1949, out-patient facilities have been extended to general hospitals in almost all areas of Egypt.

Egypt has had a Mental Health Act since 1944, which regulates the admissions and rights of mental patients. Egypt was probably the first Arab country to have such an act. This Act is centralized in that all involuntary admissions of mental patients should take place in Cairo. A new Act has been presented to parliament targeting the decentralization of psychiatric services, giving governorates full responsibility (Okasha, 1993). Although policy changes in that direction have been made, the legislation supporting them has not yet been endorsed.

Contemporary profile of mental health care services

Egypt is divided into 24 governorates, 19 with psychiatric clinics and out-patient units, and five with no psychiatric services. The latter are Matrouh, Red Sea, New Valley, and North and South Sinai.

The two largest mental hospitals in Egypt, Abbassia and Khanka, were facing great difficulties regarding care, finances, treatment, and rehabilitation while accommodating about 5,000 patients. Recently three new hospitals with 300 beds each have been built on the premises of these two hospitals with a view to providing adequate mental health services of the highest quality. The new policy of deinstitutionalization and provision of community care may reduce the number of psychiatric in-patients but will not solve the problem. Aftercare services in Egypt are still limited due to

poor understanding of the need for follow-up care after initial improvement. Community care in the form of hostels, day centres, rehabilitation
centres and health visitors is only available in big cities (Okasha and Karam,
1998). In 1967, a third mental hospital was established in Alexandria; in
1979 another was founded in Helwan; and in 1990 yet another near the air-
port. Many psychiatric units have also been established in general hospitals,
and in addition the 18 medical schools in Egypt each has a psychiatric unit
providing in-patient and out-patient psychiatric services.

The population of Egypt is 67 million. There are, approximately,
130,000 doctors, 1 for every 500 citizens; 700 psychiatrists including those
under training, 1 for every 100,000 citizens; and about 9,000 psychiatric
beds, including university, Ministry of Health and private sector hospitals
(i.e. 1 psychiatric bed for every 7,000 citizens or 15 beds per 100,000 population) (see Table 5.1). The number of psychiatric beds in Egypt constitutes less than 10% of the total number of hospital beds (110,000). Egypt
has approximately 250 clinical psychologists involved in mental health, i.e.
about 1 clinical psychologist for every 270,000 citizens. There are around
200 clinical psychologists in Cairo alone, with hundreds of general psychologists working in fields unrelated to mental health services. There are
about 300 social workers practising in psychiatric facilities (i.e. 1 social
worker for every 225,000 citizens) but unfortunately they are general social
workers with minimal graduate training in psychiatric social work. In 1960,
there was an attempt to develop the specialty of psychiatric social work at
the Institute of Social Services in Cairo. However, it lasted only two years
because of a shortage of applicants.

There are four higher institutes of nursing within Egypt – equivalent to
medical schools – that graduate highly qualified psychiatric nurses.
Unfortunately, the majority of nurses leave the country to work in the
petrodollar-rich Arabian Gulf states that pay high salaries. Most nurses
working in mental health facilities are general nurses who graduated from
nursing schools, but the numbers are insufficient to cover psychiatric services. There are about 1,355 psychiatric nurses in Egypt, 1 for every 50,000
citizens, and 900 of these are in Cairo.

Traditional and religious healers play a major role in primary psychiatric
care in Egypt. They deal with minor neurotic, psychosomatic, and transi-
tory psychotic states, using religious and group psychotherapies, sugges-
tion, and devices such as amulets and incantations (Okasha, 1966). It is estimated that 60% of out-patients at the university clinic in Cairo, serving low
socioeconomic classes, have been to traditional healers before coming to
the psychiatrist (Okasha and Karam, 1998).

Aftercare services in Egypt are still limited due to the poor understanding of most people for the need for follow-up care after an initial improvement in their health. Community care in the form of hostels, day centres,

Table 5.1 Mental health services in Egypt (MOH document 2001)

Specialty	Number	Number/Population
Doctors	130,000	1/500
Psychiatrists	700	1/100,000
Clinical Psychologists	250	1/270,000
Psychiatric Nurses	1,355	1/50,000
Social workers	300	1/225,000
MOH beds	6,400	1/10,500

rehabilitation centres, and health visitors is only available in big cities. A good example in applying community care is in the prevention of drug abuse. There has been an increase in the abuse of heroin and other narcotics since the early 1980s. The media, legislative acts, the General Administration of Drug Combat's seizures of traffickers, the initiation of centres all over Egypt and the deployment of social workers, religious people, and politicians to educate the masses about the hazards of drug abuse have all triggered an interest in psychiatry and mental disorders. Although community care started in the 1960s, active participation exploded with the increase of drug abuse among young people.

In spite of rapid social changes in Egypt, the majority of people, especially in rural areas, live in an extended family. In rural areas, community care is implemented without the need for health care workers. Egyptians, especially those living in the countryside, have a special tolerance for mental disorders and an ability to assimilate chronic mental patients. These patients, and those with mild or moderate mental retardation, are rehabilitated by cultivating and planting the countryside along with, and under the supervision of, family members. It is considered shameful not to care for an elderly demented person at home. The parents of retarded or hyperkinetic children feel a primary responsibility toward them rather than having them looked after in an institution.

Prevalence of mental disorders

Depression and anxiety disorders

The prevalence of depression among a selected sample of an urban and a rural population was found to be 11.4% and 19.7%, respectively. Dysthymic disorder was the most common diagnostic category in the urban population (4.1%) whereas adjustment disorder with depressed mood was more frequently encountered in the rural population (6.7%). Of the urban population, 1.9% were given a diagnosis of major affective disorder according to DSM-III criteria, compared with 3.3% of the rural subjects. The total prevalence was 2.5% (Okasha et al., 1988). Somatization was a common characteristic of depression. Somatic presentation seems to render mental ill-health more acceptable since psychological symptoms may be perceived culturally as a sign of lack of faith and religiosity or a weak personality, or as a characteristic mainly of females. Another study in Egypt (El Tantawy, 2000) found a prevalence of depressive disorders of 19%. Our studies revealed a higher prevalence of depression in rural than in urban areas, similar to other studies in developing countries.

A study of mental morbidity among university students in Egypt found that anxiety states were diagnosed in 36% of the total sample (Okasha et al., 1977). In 1993 anxiety states were diagnosed in about 22.6% of patients at a psychiatric out-patient clinic in a selected Egyptian sample (Okasha et al., 1993). In 1981 Okasha and Ashour undertook the first attempt to study the sociodemographic aspects of anxiety disorders in Egypt and to apply the Arabic version of the PSE (Present State Examination) in evaluating the profiles of clusters and symptoms of anxiety in a sample of 120 patients with anxiety. In a study by Okasha et al. (1999) the prevalence of anxiety symptoms in a sample of Egyptian children from three private and five public primary schools (ages 6–12 years) revealed a 7.9% prevalence of anxiety. Psychiatric co-morbidity was found in 89% of our anxiety positive sample, mainly 'behavioural and emotional disorders with onset usually occurring in childhood' and 'neurotic stress-related and somatoform disorder'. Forty per cent of children with anxiety disorders had a co-morbid depressive disorder. The findings revealed that the commonest symptoms were worrying (82%), irritability (73%), free-floating anxiety (70%), depressed mood (65%), tiredness (64%), restlessness (63%), and anergia and retardation (61%). The rarest were alcohol abuse (2%) and drug abuse (5%).

Suicide

A descriptive study of parasuicide in Cairo included 200 subjects from a total of 1,155 patients who attempted suicide in 1975. These were patients admitted to the casualty department of Ain Shams University Hospital in Cairo, which has a catchment area encompassing approximately three million people. A crude rate of suicide attempts in Cairo was found to be 38.5 per 100,000. A crude estimate of suicide in Egypt would be about 3.5 per 100,000, assuming that one in 10 suicide attempts is successful (Okasha and Lotaief, 1979).

Obsessive–compulsive disorder (OCD)

A study conducted by the Ain Shams Department of Psychiatry in 1968 on 1,000 psychiatric out-patients attending the university clinic showed an incidence of OCD of 2.5%; a replication of this study showed an incidence of 2.3%, indicating the stability of the disorder (Okasha et al., 1994).

Ninety patients suffering from OCD, diagnosed according to the *International Classification of Diseases (10th Edition)* criteria (WHO, 1992), and attending the out-patient clinic of the Institute of Psychiatry in Cairo in 1991–1992, were assessed by the Yale-Brown Obsessive–Compulsive Scale (Y-BOCS) for symptoms and severity of symptoms. The most common symptoms were religious and contamination obsessions (60%) and somatic obsessions (49%); the most common compulsions were repeating rituals (68%), cleaning and washing compulsions (63%), and checking compulsions (58%). Also, a study by Okasha et al. (2000) looked at the prevalence of obsessive–compulsive symptoms (OCS) in psychiatric patients. OCS was found to be significantly higher in various psychiatric categories than in non-psychiatric categories: 83% of patients with neurotic, stress-related and somatoform disorders, 51% of patients with mood disorders and 47% of patients with schizophrenia, schizotypal and delusional disorders were found to have OCS in their symptomatology.

In another study Okasha et al. (2001) looked at the prevalence of OCS among a community sample of Egyptian students. The prevalence of psychiatric morbidity among the total sample was 51.7%, while that of obsessive traits was 26.2% and that of obsessive–compulsive symptoms was 43.1%. OCS was more prevalent among the younger students, female students and first-born subjects. The high prevalence of OCS is secondary to the ritualistic religious upbringing in Egypt.

Policy developments

The priorities for community health care services in Egypt have traditionally not been for mental health, but rather for bilharziasis (schistosomiasis), birth control, infectious diseases in children, smoking and illicit drug abuse. Programmes for community care in big cities take the form of out-patient clinics, hostels for the elderly, institutions for the mentally retarded, and centres for drug abuse and school and university mental health.

For the years 1993–1996, the Ministry of Health budget was 1,177,226,000 Egyptian pounds, which constituted 2% of the national budget; 9% of that is assigned for mental health. The National Mental Health Programme for Egypt 1991–1996 emphasized the role of primary health care in looking after 80% of psychiatric patients. It focused on decentralization of mental health care and community care in different governorates. Emphasis was on recruiting mental health teams, especially psychiatric nurses, psychiatric social workers, occupational therapists and clinical psychologists.

The new National Mental Health Programme for the years 1997–2002 was drafted within a general health sector reform in Egypt. The Egyptian Ministry of Health defined the Health Sector Reform Programme as a health system that assures universal coverage to the population through a basic package of health services, and should be based on the principles of equity, efficiency, quality, affordability, sustainability and client satisfaction. The aim of the programme was for the expectation of a disability-free life for all. Components of the reform included health care service reform, human resource reform, health sector infrastructure reform, institutional development, health care financing reform and pharmaceutical reform. It was agreed that the success of the project should rely on primary health care to achieve acceptable levels of health for all, emphasize the importance of disease prevention and health promotion, and focus on family medicine with an emphasis on family doctor training.

Mental health has been acknowledged by the programme as a vital component of health, based on its important role in the development of Egypt. Objectives of the mental health sector reform included:

- Increasing productivity.
- Decreasing long hospital stay.
- Decreasing expenditure on expensive drugs.
- Alleviation of a significant part of the direct and indirect costs to society in general.

The reform programme targets Ministry of Health (MOH) hospitals and clinics, university hospitals and clinics, non-governmental organizations, private hospitals and clinics, and the health facilities of the defence and interior ministries.

The mental health policy and strategy in Egypt relies basically on co-operation between the Ministry of Health and other concerned ministries. It aims to establish preventive and promotional activities in the field of mental health, to introduce an effective mental health programme in primary health care, to reduce overall costs, and to put special emphasis on health and social policies designed to enhance mental development. Priority areas include primary health care services, prevention and early detection, rehabilitation and the development of health management information systems and surveillance.

Its goals were formulated as follows:

- To enhance the awareness of mental health at different levels.
- To prevent mental disorders mainly in vulnerable groups.
- To manage people with mental disorders or addiction problems in a qualified manner.
- To emphasize rehabilitation as an important and effective method for preventing relapses and disability.

Improvement of resources for the implementation of the programme is to be achieved through strengthening the utilization of human resources, reallocation of some resources towards rehabilitation and intermediate services, improving treatment practices, developing mental health services as an integral part of primary health care services, introducing community-based practices, and focusing more attention on promotion of mental welfare in society. It is expected that family health care could play an important role in the prevention and early detection of mental problems, the diagnosis and treatment of non-advanced mentally ill patients, and the referral of more advanced cases to psychiatrists. This would require the sensitive deployment of primary health care providers properly trained in the recognition and treatment of mental disorders, and the upgrading of mental health services as a backup to first-line workers.

This approach would require a shift in focus from hospital-based mental health care to out-patient-based care. The focus would be on the mental health care of children and adolescents, paying special attention to school health, and the recognition of mental health by policymakers as a part of the basic benefits package.

The Ministry of Health has committed itself to allocating more resources to develop and maintain the physical structure of mental health care institutions, and to increasing the number of mental hospital beds. At present the mental health budget constitutes about 8% of the total health budget, which is still below the minimum of 10% recommended by the World Health Organization. The Ministry of Health spending on mental health services has increased from $14 million to $17.8 million in the last three years. Although this can be taken as a positive indicator, the implementation of the mental health programme does not continue unchallenged.

Primary evaluations of the reform process have pointed to some of those difficulties:

- An increase in patient expenditure from $5.2 million in 1998–1999 to $9.2 million in 2000–2001 because of the high cost of mental health medications.
- A huge increase in the annual cost per admission from $1,425 in 1997–1998 to $2,650 in 1999–2000 due to the increase in expenditure for expensive medication.
- Approximately a doubling in the cost per bed from $1,100 in 1997–1998 to $2,168 in 1990–2000.

The universal process of globalization tends towards the privatization of basic services and the withdrawal of the state as a provider or supporter of such services.

Managed care in psychiatry has been one product of the globalization policy in the health sector. For southern countries like Egypt, managed care will call for a system of mental health personnel consisting of psychiatrists, clinical psychologists, psychiatric social workers, nurses and counsellors. It will need a good referral system and adequate training for primary care physicians who are skilled in filtering, referring, diagnosing and managing patients with mental disorders. The cost-saving policy will come heavy with its own cost requirements and will put extra burden on policymakers and mental health providers (Okasha, 1999b).

Agreements with the World Trade Organization will eventually lead to an even greater increase of the cost of medications, expected to be beyond the purchase ability of the majority of the population. At the same time the prevalence of mental disorders, foremost depression, substance abuse and the detection of childhood mental disorders, are expected to rise, putting a greater demand on the mental health care system. Maintaining the balance between resources and demand, without violating citizens' rights to equal access to mental health care, will be a challenge.

Homosexuality

During the XI World Congress of Psychiatry in Hamburg 1999, there was a debate about homosexuality. The American Psychiatric Association presented a statement to be endorsed by the general assembly that homosexuality, since it is not now considered a mental disorder in international classifications, should be removed from all textbooks where it is classed as such. Many delegates, especially from traditional societies, debated the subject and stated that in their societies homosexuality is considered a sin and should be punished. The only escape from stigma is to label it a mental disorder. In spite of the endorsement of the declaration of human rights by all countries of the world that there should be no discrimination because of sexual inclination, many countries do not abide by the resolution.

Recently, in Egypt, 50 young people who were cruising in a boat on the Nile were arrested and indicted for practising sinful acts including homosexuality and worshipping devils. They were not referred to the ordinary judiciary system but to a special security court which rules according to emergency laws. These people denied the accusations and claimed that they were having an ordinary party. They were subjected to forensic examination to look for evidence of sodomy. The trial created much media debate, but the majority of the population condemned the defendants even before the verdict of the trial. Many human rights activists blamed the situation of human rights in Egypt, but they were ridiculed by the mass media for being under Western influence, which, the media claimed, encourages sexual perversion against the teachings of all religions.

A number of the accused were punished by several years of imprisonment. However, international and national pressure from campaigns by human rights activists succeeded, and the President of the Republic has used his constitutional authority to stop the enactment of the court ruling and has ordered a re-trial. This is an example of a conflict between traditional, psychiatric and political judgement of a social phenomenon that challenges psychiatrists and their societies to take a position.

Conclusion

The growing financial resources allocated in many countries to the providers of health care, and the calls for controls on health care expenditure, suggest a need for a consideration of the repercussions of mental illness across society, the costs related to health care provision and the health and economic return due to care and assistance.

There are several major issues in measuring the economic cost of mental illness that are potentially large in magnitude and controversial in their conclusions. These are the costs to families of care of a mentally ill member, co-morbidity costs, capital costs, labour market impact of mental illness and non-productivity losses due to illness. Other costs are those associated with improper measurements, unreliable diagnostic systems and inappropriate measures of reliability. These costs are felt when resources and talents are used in a wasteful fashion and misleading information leads to inappropriate research (Bartko, 1990). The extent of these costs depend on several factors: the duration of the disease, the level of impairment caused, the type of specialized service required, the age of onset, and the duration of the disorder. Finally the total costs to society depend on the size of the population affected by the disorder.

Physicians, policymakers and others active in the health care systems around the world continue to struggle to maintain a balance between the need to contain costs, and efforts to maintain or improve both access to services and the quality of care provided.

In the last few years a number of research studies have attempted to identify factors related to psychiatric costs, not only to achieve a more cost-effective deployment of resources but also to develop a funding system better tailored to community-based psychiatric services.

Reduction of cost for health care and a more effective use of resources could speed up the provision of services to many who at present do not have access to appropriate treatment. While there is general agreement about the desirability of a more rational use of resources, there is little certainty that the methods necessary for an economic analysis of mental health programmes are sufficiently developed to be recommended for general application.

Despite all economic constraints, the importance of setting a minimum of expenditure on health, cannot be over-emphasized to ensure the proper planning and allocation of resources. While the total health budget represents 7–14% of the gross national product in industrial countries, it ranges from 1–5% in the developing countries. The World Bank has estimated that 80% of the total health budget in the world is spent on 10% of the population, and 20% of the total health budget in the world is spent on 90% of the population, with a health budget for individuals ranging from $3,500 in the USA to $1 in some countries. The irony is that over 80% of the weapons deals and weapons supplies, which directly contribute to the instability and violence in the world, are by the five permanent members of the Security Council.

Yet, despite the recognized need for cost containment, clinicians, policymakers and consumers should be concerned that this could adversely affect quality or outcomes of care, especially for vulnerable populations such as those with serious psychiatric disorders. On the basis of world statistics the solution may be found in resource allocation rather than health cost containment. The involvement of consumers in the planning and monitoring process of health policy development may be a first step in that direction.

References

Baasher T (1975) The Arab countries. In Howells TG (Ed.) World History of Psychiatry. NY and London: Churchill Livingstone.

Bartko JJ (1990) Measurement and reliability: Statistical thinking considerations. First Workshop on Costs and Assessment in Psychiatry. The Cost of Schizophrenia, Venice, October 29–31.

Burgel JC (1972) Psychosomatic Methods, 163; idem, Der Mufarrih an-nafs des Ibn Qadi Ba'albakk, ein Lehrbuch der Psychohygiene aus dem 7. Jahrhundert der Hijra, in Proceedings of the Sixth Congress of Arabic and Islamic studies, Leiden 1975, p. 204.

Dols MW (1992) Majnun: The Madman in Medieval Islamic Society. Immisch DE (Ed.) Oxford: Clarendon Press.

El Tantawy A (1998) An epidemiological study of depressive disorders in Ismailia governorate Egypt. MD Thesis, Suez Canal University .

Ministry of Health (1998) Statistics. Cairo: Ministry of Health.

Ministry of Health (2001) Statistics. Cairo: Ministry of Health.

National Institute of Planning (1998) Human development report – Egypt. Cairo: National Institute of Planning.

Okasha A (1966) A cultural psychiatric study of El Zar Cult in UAR. British Journal of Psychiatry, 160(Suppl. 16): 4–72.

Okasha A (1988) Clinical Psychiatry. Cairo: Anglo-Egyptian Bookshop.

Okasha A (1993) Psychiatry in Egypt. British Journal of Psychiatry, 17: 548–51.

Okasha A (1999a) Challenges of Managed Mental Health Care in the South East Mediterranean Region. In Guimon J, Sartorius N (Eds.) Manage or Perish. New York: Kluwer Academic.

Okasha A (1999b) Mental Health in the Middle East: An Egyptian Perspective. Clinical Psychology Review, 19(8): 917–33.

Okasha A, Ashou C (1981) Psychodemographic study of anxiety in Egypt. The PSE in its Arabic version. British Journal of Psychiatry 139: 70.

Okasha A, Hassan A (1968) Preliminary psychiatric observations in Egypt. British Journal of Psychiatry, 114(513): 949–55.

Okasha A, Karam E (1998) Mental health services and research in the Arab world. Acta Psychiatrica Scandinavica, 98: 406–13.

Okasha A, Lotaief F (1979) Attempted suicide: An Egyptian investigation. Acta Psychiatrica Scandinavica, 60: 69.

Okasha A, Okasha T (2000) Mental health in Cairo (Al-Qahira). International Journal of Mental Health, 28(4): 62–8.

Okasha A, Kamel M, Sadek A, Lotaief F, Bishry Z (1977) Psychiatric morbidity among university students in Egypt. British Journal of Psychiatry, 131: 149.

Okasha A, Khalil AH, El Fiky MR, Ghanem M, Abdel Hakeem R (1988) Prevalence of depressive disorder in a sample of rural and urban Egyptian communities. Egyptian Journal of Psychiatry, 2: 167.

Okasha A, Seif El Dawla A, Assad A (1993) Presentation of hysteria in a sample of Egyptian patients – An update. Neurology, Psychiatry, and Brain Research, 1: 155.

Okasha A, Saad A, Khalil AH, Seif El Dawla A, Yehia N (1994) Phenomenology of OCD: A transcultural study. Comprehensive Psychiatry, 35(3): 191.

Okasha A, Bishry Z, Seif El Dawla A, Saye M, Okasha T (1999) Prevalence of anxiety symptoms in a sample of Egyptian children. Current Psychiatry, 6(3): 356–68.

Okasha A, Lotaief F, Ashour AM, El Mahalawy N, Seif El Dawla A, El Kholy GH (2000) The prevalence of obsessive–compulsive symptoms in a sample of Egyptian psychiatric patients. L'Encephale, XXVI: 1–10.

Okasha A, Ragheb K, Attia AH, Seif El Dawla A, Okasha T, Imail R (2001) Prevalence of obsessive–compulsive symptoms (OCS) in a sample of Egyptian adolescents. L'Encephale, XXVII: 8–14.

Statistical Year Book (1997) Cairo: National Information Centre.

Warnock J, Dudgeon HW (1920) Report for the Year 1920. Ministry of Interior, Egypt, Lunacy Division. Cairo: Government Press.

World Health Organization (1992) International Classification of Diseases (10th edition). WHO: Geneva.

CHAPTER SIX

India: Towards community mental health care

R. SRINIVASA MURTHY

Introduction

India enters the 21st century with many changes in the social, political, economic and scientific fields. There is both a reconsideration of social institutions and reorganization of policies and programmes (e.g. National Health Policy, 2002). The mental health scene in India, during recent years, reflects the complexity of an evolving mental health policy in a developing country. During this period, there has been a critical examination of existing mental hospitals in the country. First, the human rights point of view has been examined by the National Human Rights Commission of India (NHRC, 1999). Second, the Supreme Court of India is continuously examining a wide variety of issues relating to mental health care following the Erwadi tragedy in which 28 mentally ill persons were burned to death in an accidental fire while chained to pillars (Frontline, 2001). Third, the National Health Policy (2002) clearly spells out the place of mental health in the overall planning of health care.

These recent developments have occurred against the background of over 25 years of: efforts to integrate mental health care with primary health care (from 1975); replacement of the Indian Lunacy Act 1912 by the Mental Health Act 1987; and the enactment of the Persons with Disabilities Act 1995, focusing on the equal opportunities, protection of rights and full participation of disabled persons. The main challenges for developing a mental health policy in India are: the extremely limited number of mental health professionals (about 10,000 professionals of all categories for one billion population); the very limited mental health service infrastructure (about 30,000 psychiatric beds for a billion population); limited investment in health by the government (estimated public sector expenditure on health is only 13% of total health expenditure); problems of poverty (about 30% of the population live below the poverty line); and literacy levels of only around 60%, with much lower rates among women.

This review of mental health policy in India covers: (1) historical aspects of the development of mental health care; (2) the development of the National Mental Health Programme since 1982; (3) Mental Health Act, 1987 and the Persons with Disabilities Act, 1995; (4) progress of the National Mental Health Programme; (5) the Report of the National Human Rights Commission on the State of the Mental Hospitals in India; (6) the Erwadi tragedy on 6 August 2001; (7) the initiatives of the Supreme Court regarding mental health legislation, human rights and mental health care since August 2001; (8) mental health plans during the 10th Five Year Plan (2002–2007); (9) National Health Policy (2002); and (10) strengths and weaknesses of the mental health policies.

Historical aspects of mental health care

In India a highly developed and elaborate system of medicine has flourished for nearly 3,000 years. It is generally known by the name of *Ayurveda* [the science of life]. There are many medical texts dating back to the 1st and 2nd centuries AD which describe in detail the principles of *Ayurveda*. The two best-known medical works are by the Ayurvedic physicians Caraka and Susruta. These books were originally compiled some time between the 3rd century BC and the 3rd century AD. The principles of Ayurvedic medicine, as in other Indian philosophical systems, were probably well developed by the 3rd century BC. All the major Ayurvedic texts, such as Carak Samhita and Susruta Simhata, have separate sections dealing with insanity [*unmada*]. In addition, there are chapters on spirit possession [*bhutonmada*] and epilepsy [*apasmara*]. Different types of convulsions, paralysis, fainting and intoxications are also well described. There are detailed descriptions of different types of spirit possessions. Although at times the descriptions appear artificial, some of them have clear resemblance to some modern descriptions of personality disorders, psychosis, and mental retardation. The chapters on *unmada* [insanity] are very detailed, both in Caraka Samhita and Susruta Samhita (Srinivasa Murthy and Wig, 2002).

The growth of asylums in India until independence is well reviewed by Bhugra (2001). The salient features of this period are taken from his exhaustive review. Although there is an occasional mention of asylums in ancient India, the last known asylums existed in the 9th century AD in Madras (Bhugra, 2001; Somasundaram, 1973). The initial history of psychiatry in India is argued to be the history of the establishment of mental hospitals and the occasional increase in their accommodation as need demanded (Varma, 1953). Although Western-style hospitals and medicine were introduced in India by the Portuguese, it was the British who established the asylums. The early establishment of mental hospitals in the Indian subcontinent is said to have reflected the needs and demands of European patients in India. Initially, these were in Calcutta, Madras and Bombay – cities that were growing with British influence and expertise. One of the British leaders of that period, Shaw (1932), held a very strong view that Europeans and persons of European habits should not, as a rule, be treated in the same mental hospitals as Indians; not on any grounds of sentiment, but because the accommodation and amenities necessary for the one are unsuited to the other.

Since independence

During the last 55 years, the place of mental health as part of the general health system has changed significantly. From a situation of no organized mental health care at the time of independence, currently, mental health issues are seen as part of the public agenda in various forms. A reflection of this is the clear reference to mental health in the National Health Policy (2002) and the nine-fold increase in public health allocation for the mental health programme during the next five years. The overall effect has been the recognition of mental health as an important issue in the community, and the movement of services from mental hospital care to care in the community. Mental health professionals in India have viewed community mental health not as care in the community but care utilizing community resources – in other words care *by* the community.

Beginning with the report of the Bhore Health Survey and Development Committee (Bhore, 1946), mental health has been part of general health planning in the country. The Bhore Committee observed:

> Even if the proportion of patients be taken as 2 per 1,000 population in India, hospital accommodation should be available for at least 800,000 mental patients as against the existing provision for a little over 10,000 beds for the country as a whole.
>
> (Bhore, 1946: 130)

The proposals from the Bhore Committee for mental health care were (1) the creation of mental health organizations as part of the establishments under the Director General of Health Services at the centre and of the Provincial Directors of Health Services; (2) the improvement of the existing 17 mental hospitals and the establishment of two new institutions in the first five years, and of five more during the next five years; (3) the provision of facilities for training in mental health work for medical staff in India and abroad, and for ancillary personnel in India; and (4) the establishment of a Department of Mental Health in the proposed All India Medical Institute, New Delhi.

The next Health Review Committee to examine the health situation in the country was the Mudaliar Committee in 1962. This Committee assessed the progress made subsequent to the Bhore Committee, that is, in the intervening two decades, as follows:

Reliable statistics regarding the incidence of mental morbidity in India are not available. It is believed that enormous numbers of patients require psychiatric assistance and service. As against the total need, the number of beds available in mental hospitals in India is only 15,000.

(Mudaliar, 1962: 6)

The recommendations in the report of the Mudaliar Committee were: (1) to set up in-patient departments at lay hospitals, independent psychiatric clinics, mental health clinics, and institutions for mental defectives; (2) to train personnel in mental health, with orientation in mental hygiene for all medical and health personnel, and in particular pediatricians, schoolteachers, nurses and administrators; (3) to deal with the acute shortage of psychiatrists by upgrading the Ranchi Mental Hospital into a fully fledged training institution in addition to the All India Institute of Mental Health, Bangalore; (4) to arrange that, ultimately, each region, if not each state, become self-sufficient in training its total requirement of mental health personnel.

An important outcome of this Committee's recommendations was the setting up of a number of district psychiatric units in different parts of the country and the creation of a mental health advisory group at the Ministry of Health.

These two reports are important as they represent the aspirations of the policymakers at the time, and progress can be measured against the goals set early in independent India.

The National Health Policy (1983) provided a new direction for health planning in India. One of the main recommendations was the increased emphasis on community participation and empowerment of the community for health. However, the National Health Policy of 1983 refers to mental health care only indirectly, as follows:

Special well-coordinated programmes should be launched to provide mental health care as well as medical care and also the physical and social rehabilitation of those who are mentally retarded, deaf, dumb, blind, physically disabled, infirm, and the aged.

(National Health Policy, 1983: 9)

In the first 30 years (1947–1975) the main focus was to develop centres of training for psychiatrists, clinical psychologists, psychiatric social workers and psychiatric nurses; to shift care to general hospital psychiatric units (Wig, 1978); and to involve families in care.

From 1975 to 1981, two systematic efforts to integrate mental health with primary health care were initiated at Bangalore and Chandigarh. This effort involved: (1) understanding of the needs of mentally ill persons in the community (Chandrasekar et al., 1981; Issac and Kapur, 1980; Issac et al., 1981, 1982; Parthasarathy et al., 1981; Srinivasa Murthy et al., 1974, 1976, 1978; Wig et al., 1980, 1981a); (2) understanding the needs of mentally ill persons attending general health facilities (Harding et al., 1980; Shamasunder et al., 1983; Seshadri et al., 1988; Srinivasa Murthy et al., 1976); (3) developing psychiatric training manuals (Issac et al., 1988; Sell et al., 1989; Shamasunder et al., 1983, 1986; Srinivasa Murthy et al., 1988; Sriram et al., 1991; Wig and Srinivasa Murthy, 1980) for training the different categories of health personnel and for evaluating the impact of the training (Menon et al., 1978; Nagarajiah et al., 1994; Shamasunder et al., 1983, 1986; Sriram et al., 1987, 1989, 1990a, 1990b, 1990c); and (4) the care provided (Wig et al., 1981b).

These efforts led to the development of a National Mental Health Programme (NMHP, 1982). The launching of this programme is a milestone in mental health planning in India. The document was presented to the Central Council of Health and Family Welfare (CCHFW), the highest policymaking body in the area of health, at its meeting in August 1982. The group made the following recommendations:

> Mental health must form an integral part of the total health programme and as such should be included in all national policies and programmes in the field of health, education and social welfare and, realizing the importance of mental health in the course curricula for various levels of health professionals, suitable action should be taken in consultation with the appropriate authorities to strengthen the mental health component.
>
> (CCHFW, 1982: 15)

The objectives of the National Mental Health Programme (1982) were:

1. To ensure availability and accessibility of minimum mental health care for all in the foreseeable future, particularly to the most vulnerable and underprivileged of the population.
2. To encourage application of mental health knowledge in general health care and in social development.
3. To promote community participation in mental health service development and to stimulate effort towards self-help in the community.

The specific approaches suggested for the implementation of the NMHP were: diffusion of mental health skills to the periphery of the health service system; appropriate appointment of tasks in mental health care; equitable and balanced territorial distribution of resources; integration of basic mental health care with general health services; and linkage to community development.

Since the formulation of the NMHP in August 1982 many initiatives and activities have been taken up to implement the programme. For example: raising the level of awareness, about mental health, of the state level programme officers, and gaining their involvement; workshops for voluntary agencies and mental health professionals, namely psychiatrists, clinical psychologists, psychiatric social workers, and psychiatric nurses; training programmes in public mental health for programme managers; development of models of integration of mental health into primary health care up to the level of the district (1–2 million population); preparation of support materials in the form of health education manuals for different types of health personnel; training programmes for the teachers of undergraduate psychiatry; extension of the district programme to 25 districts; and setting standards for mental hospitals and support to voluntary organizations for mental health initiatives.

These developments were the result of efforts by a large group of mental health professionals taking up the various issues relating to mental health at different centres (Gautam, 1985; Satyavathi, 1993; Sharma, 1986; Wig and Parhee, 1984). A very important area of ongoing research is the study of mental disorders in primary health care (Amin et al., 1998; Channabasavanna et al., 1995; Chisholm et al., 2000; Manickam, 1997; Patel, 2000; Patel et al., 1998; Pereira and Patel, 1998; Sen, 1987; Srinivasa Murthy et al., 1976).

Of the many initiatives, the integration of mental health with primary health care at the level of the district is the most important. The approach of this initiative was intensive community-based mental health care. The principles of the District Mental Health Programme, as developed at the Bellary district, were:

- a decentralized training programme for the existing health personnel on essentials of mental health care at the district level;
- provision of mental health care in all general health facilities;
- involvement of all categories of health and welfare personnel in mental health care;
- provision of essential psychiatric drugs at all health facilities;
- a simple system of record keeping;
- a mechanism to monitor the work of primary health care personnel in the provision of mental health care;
- a mental health team at the district level for training personnel, referral support and supervision of the mental health programme.

The initial project at Bellary demonstrated the feasibility of providing basic mental health care along with primary health care (Issac 1986; Naik et al., 1994, 1996). However, there is no specific schedule to take up the programme on a wider scale for the next five years. Since 1995, the District

Mental Health Programme has been launched at the national level. A budgetary allocation of Rs. 28.00 crores was made during the Ninth Five Year Plan period (1995–2000) for the National Mental Health Programme. The goal here was:

> A community-based approach to the problem, which includes (1) training of the mental health team at the identified nodal institutes within the state; (2) increasing awareness in the care necessity about mental health problems; (3) providing services for early detection and treatment of mental illness in the community itself with both OPD [out-patient department] and indoor treatment and follow-up of discharged cases; and provide valuable data and experience at the level of community in the state and centre for future planning improvement in service and research. The training of trainers at the state level is being provided regularly by the National Institute of Mental Health and Neurosciences, Bangalore under the NMHP.
>
> (GOI, 2000)

The DMHP was extended to seven districts in 1997–1998, a further five districts in 1998, and six more districts in 1999–2000. Currently the programme is under implementation in 25 districts within 20 states.

Progress of the National Mental Health Programme

The Sixth Conference of the CCHFW, held in April 1999, noted that:

> Mental health problems are on the increase and this has been a neglected area so far. The Council appreciated the efforts of the Ministry of Health in initiating pilot projects in the area of community mental health through the District Mental Health Programme (DMHP) in some states. It recommends that more state governments should take advantage of the various training programmes to create more trained manpower at the periphery and at the grass root level, and more states and UTs [union territories] should actively participate in the DMHP. The Council notes with concern the unhygienic and inhuman environment in some of the mental hospitals and recommends that mental hospitals adopt prescribed minimum standards of care for this purpose. In view of the increasing demand for psychiatric services in rural areas, the Council urges that the medical Council of India examine and upgrade the training curriculum in psychiatry at the undergraduate level in medical colleges, if necessary by making it a compulsory subject. The Council further recommends that more focused attention be paid to establishing counselling facilities for handling vulnerable categories suffering from mental stress due to (1) poverty ... domestic violence; (2) aged; (3) children and adolescents; and (4) victims of natural and man-made calamities and disasters. The other recommendations for action are to initiate information, education and communication activities for public education using all media and monitoring and evaluation mechanisms for mental health programmes. (CCHFW, 1999: 23)

A meeting in October 2000, of policymakers and mental health professionals reviewed the progress of the DMHP. Its aims were to consider the impediments and bottlenecks, to identify mid-course corrections, and to develop strategies for expanding the DMHP in the country. The review identified the following issues in the implementation of DMHP: (1) a lack of administrative clarity to utilize allocated funds; (2) difficulty in recruiting staff; (3) the need for a central co-ordinating committee; (4) training needs of DMHP staff; (5) revision of the manuals for training of primary health care staff; (6) widening the scope of activities of the DMHP; and (7) development of indicators to monitor the programme.

The review group recommended that the DMHP should be extended in a phased manner, and that central co-ordinating and supporting mechanisms should be instituted. It also suggested that there was a need to develop clearer guidelines for financial matters, and for inspection of the programme periodically at local, state and national levels. The activities for mental health care should, the group advocated, include common mental disorders, rehabilitation, public mental health education, and primary prevention. The inclusion of private general practitioners was recognized as relevant. The development of simple training modules for family members was regarded as important.

The review group noted the needs of the growing urban population which need to be addressed. The other activities identified for further work were the development of information, education and communication (IEC) materials, revision of the manuals, and the development of a network of professionals working with the DMHP. There was also concern for the sustenance of the programme beyond the five year period of support from the Centre.

Legislative initiatives

In keeping with other changes, the Indian Lunacy Act (1912) was replaced by a more appropriate Mental Health Act in 1987. The new Act has a variety of admission procedures to decrease the need for judicial admissions, and in relation to the discharge of patients, a system of licensing to maintain standards of mental health care. The protection of human rights of the mentally ill individual is presented as follows:

> Section 81. No mentally ill person shall be subjected during treatment to any indignity (whether physical or mental) or cruelty; no mentally ill person under treatment shall be used for purposes of research unless (1) such research is of direct benefit to him for purposes of diagnosis or treatment or (2) such person, being a voluntary patient, has given his consent in writing or

where such person (whether or not a voluntary patient) is incompetent, by reason of minority or otherwise, to give valid consent, the guardian or other person competent to give consent on his behalf, has given his consent in writing, for such research ... no letters or other communications sent by or to mentally ill persons under treatment shall be intercepted, detained or destroyed.

(Mental Health Act 1987: 31)

Another important provision is the establishment of a Mental Health Authority at central and state levels to regulate, develop, direct and co-ordinate mental health services, and to supervise the psychiatric hospitals, psychiatric nursing homes and other mental health service agencies.

The rules for implementation of the Mental Health Act were formulated in December 1990. The initial reaction was objection by the professionals to the system of licensing. However, since none of the states took up the provisions of the Act, there was no serious opposition to it. Consequently, the full implementation of the Mental Health Act 1987 has not occurred. However, the Erwadi Tragedy (Frontline, 2001) brought into focus the dangers of unregulated institutional mental health care. Following the tragedy, the non-implementation of the Act to regulate services is one of the issues in front of the Supreme Court of India at present. Along with this focus on the implementation of the Act, private psychiatrists have raised many objections about the Act and have called for a total revision of the Act or the formulation of a new Act. The objections are that the Act suffers from a number of inherent infirmities, defects, lacunae, and in certain parts, is totally unimplementable. The Act is thought to fail to address the real needs of mental health care and to contribute to stigma, isolation and discrimination of people with mental disorders. One of the serious limitations of the Act and the Rules is the single norm for licensing of psychiatric facilities, without recognizing the variety of settings in which people with mental disorders are provided care. The other objection is the non-availability of personnel to staff the facilities as per the Act.

The Persons with Disabilities Act (1995) covers the equal opportunities, protection of rights and full participation of people with disabilities. Among the different categories of disabled, 'mental illness' is included. In the last seven years since the law has been in force, major developments to provide welfare benefits, create reserved employment, create barrier-free environments, and set up local level groups to support the disabled have been initiated. The law has been a great catalyst for the improvement of the lives of the disabled. However, not all the benefits are being applied to mentally disabled people. To date, the certification process to categorize the degree of disability has been finalized for all other disabilities except mental disorders.

The 1999 NHRC report on the state of mental hospitals in India

The 1999 NHRC report is a monumental effort to document systematically the current situation of mental hospitals. That it was such an effort, and that it was urgently needed, can be made out by the following quotations from the findings of the report, which relate to 37 government psychiatric hospitals:

> Thirty-eight per cent of the hospitals still retain the jail-like structure they had at the time of inception ... nine of the hospitals constructed before 1900 have a custodial type of architecture, compared to four built during pre-independence and one post-independence ... 57% have high walls ... patients are referred to as 'inmates' and persons in whose care the patients remain through most of the day are referred to as 'warders' and their supervisors as 'overseers' and the different wards are referred to as 'enclosures' (p. 32) ... overcrowding in large hospitals was evident (p. 34) ... the overall ratio of cots:patient is 1:1.4 indicating that floor beds are a common occurrence in many hospitals (p. 37) ... in hospitals at Varanasi, Indore, Murshadabad and Ahmedabad patients are expected to urinate and defecate into open drains in public view (p. 38) ... many hospitals have problems with running water ... water storage facilities are also poor in 70% of hospitals ... lighting is inadequate in 38% of the hospitals ... 89% had closed wards while 51% had exclusively closed wards ... 43% have cells for isolation of patients (p. 39) ... leaking roofs, overflowing toilets, eroded floors, broken doors and windows are common sights (p. 44) ... privacy for patients was present in less than half the hospitals ... seclusion rooms were present in 76% of hospitals and used in the majority of these hospitals ... only 14% of the staff felt that their hospital inpatient facility was adequate (p. 47) ... in most hospitals case file recording was extremely inadequate ... less than half of the hospitals have clinical psychologists and psychiatric social workers ... trained psychiatric nurses were present in less than 25% of the hospitals (p. 48) ... even routine blood and urine tests were not available in more than 20% of hospitals ... 81% of those in charge of the mental hospitals reported that their staff position was inadequate (p. 54).
>
> (NHRC, 1999)

This was the situation in 1999, somewhat similar to the situation in hospitals in Western countries at the end of the 19th century. The report notes, 'The deficiencies in the areas described so far are enough indicators that the rights of the mentally ill are grossly violated in mental hospitals' (p. 50).

As recommended by the National Human Rights Commission, there is an urgent and massive need for change in the situation relating to mental hospitals. They need to become centres of care and treatment rather than custodial institutions.

The Erwadi tragedy in August 2001

An unfortunate incident has highlighted the lack of meaningful services and the lack of regulation of mental health care facilities. On 6 August 2001, 28 persons perished in an accidental fire while chained to pillars in Erwadi, Tamil Nadu. This tragic outcome stems from an all-too-common practice of relatives of 'chronic' patients seeking solutions in religious centres, believed to be associated with healing powers, mainly due to lack of alternatives. At the time of the tragedy more than 400 persons with various mental disorders were housed in about 20 houses in the town of Erwadi. These houses were under the care of lay persons and there was no medical care available. Fire broke out in one of the houses and those chained to the pillars perished. The incident created an uproar among the public, and the media seized the occasion to focus not only on the plight of the Erwadi patients but also on the thousands of similar cases in different parts of the country.

The Erwadi incident has resulted in Parliament debating the issue, the Supreme Court taking up the rights of mentally ill people by asking for reports from each of the states in the country, and the NHRC initiating an independent inquiry into the matter. All the centres of custodial care with no professional support have been ordered to close. Many of the patients have been sent home or shifted to treatment centres. Psychiatrists have been appointed in all the 25 districts, an increase from 14 prior to the incident. It is expected that standards of care and a system of licensing of centres for treatment will come into force as envisaged in the Mental Health Act 1987.

The state of Tamil Nadu, in which the tragedy occurred, set up a commission to review mental health care in the state and suggested comprehensive plans for mental health care. The commission presented its report to the state legislature on 30 November 2002. The recommendations included:

> Setting up of mental hospitals in Thanjavur, Tiruchi, Madurai and Ramanathapuram, and one of them exclusively for women. Currently, the state has only one mental hospital in Chennai and the relatives of patients from distant places find it difficult to bring them to Chennai. The commission has recommended that a psychiatrist be posted in every district hospital; it has also stressed the need to set up a psychiatric clinic in every district headquarters and a 10-bed psychiatric ward in major hospitals. Concessions of the sort extended to the physically challenged, the commission said, should be extended to the mentally challenged too. It urged the government to monitor all places of worship that house the mentally ill and to close down unlicensed private asylums.
>
> (Frontline, 2002: 132).

Another important outcome is in the district of Ramanathapuram, where Erwadi is located. The district administration took a series of measures to deal with the situation, including the setting up of satellite mental health centres, identifying the mentally ill by organizing camps in various places, and providing vocational and community-based rehabilitation. It set up a medical review team, which visits the satellite mental health centres every month to follow up one the patients identified.

Court initiatives regarding mental health legislation, human rights and mental health care

State level high courts and the national level Supreme Court of India have stepped in to address the human rights of mentally ill persons during the last 20 years. There has been public interest litigation to address the abuse of mentally ill persons in the mental hospitals of Trivandrum, Poona, Ranchi, Gwalior, Agra, and Delhi (AIR, 1995a, 1995b; Supreme Court Commission Report, 1984). In all these cases improvements have been made in the institutions. In 1993, the issue of gaoling the mentally ill as 'non-crimnal lunatics' in the states of West Bengal and Assam was taken up, and the court directed abolition of the practice of admitting non-criminal mentally ill people to gaol (Dhanda, 2000; Supreme Court Commission Report 1984). Directions from the judgment of the Supreme Court in the Sheela Barse vs. West Bengal case (Dhanda, 2000) referred to the need for comprehensive mental health care, which included:

> Immediate upgradation of mental hospitals ... Setting up of psychiatric services in all teaching and district hospitals ... Integrating mental health care with the primary health care system.

The Erwadi tragedy in 2001 has brought to focus the needs of people with mental disorders and their families (Frontline, 2001). Since August 2001, the Supreme Court has been examining the issues and periodically providing directions for change.

In its interim order dated 5 February 2002, the Supreme Court directed:

> Every state and union territory must undertake a district-wide survey of all registered/unregistered bodies, by whatever name called, purporting to offer psychiatric/mental health care. All such bodies should be granted or refused licence depending upon whether minimum prescribed standards are fulfilled ... Both the central and state governments shall undertake a comprehensive awareness campaign with a special rural focus to educate people as to provisions of law [regarding] mental health, rights of mentally challenged persons, the fact that chaining of mentally challenged persons is illegal and that mental patients should be sent to doctors and not to religious places such as temples or dargahs.

In continuation of the order dated 5 February 2002, on 17 April 2002, the Supreme Court further directed:

> Considering various provisions of the Mental Health Act, 1987, particularly Section 5 which inter alia provides that central government may in any part of India, or state government may, within the limits of its jurisdiction, establish or maintain psychiatric hospitals or psychiatric nursing homes for the admission, treatment and care of mentally ill persons at such places as it thinks fit. It is directed as under: 1. Every state and union territory (UT) shall undertake a comprehensive need assessment survey and file the report thereof on the following aspects: (a) estimated availability of mental health resource personnel in the state, including psychiatrists, psychologists, psychiatric social workers and psychiatric nurses in both the public and private (licensed) sector; (b) type of mental health delivery system available in the state, including the available bed strength, outpatient services and rehabilitation services in the public and private (licensed) sector; (c) an estimate of the mental health services (including personnel and facilities) that would be required, having regard to the population of the state and the incidence of mental illness.

The 5 February 2002 and 17 April 2002 directions of the Supreme Court are path breaking in demanding a greater accountability of the state towards mentally ill persons. However, the specific measures are limited and there is a need to develop a broader mental health agenda for India. The focus on institutionalized people would mean that only about one in 100 with severe mental disorders will be provided relief by the steps outlined by the Supreme Court. The instruction to set up immediately a mental hospital would direct resources to buildings and other facilities rather than organizing the larger community-based and decentralized mental health care envisaged by the National Health Policy 2002.

The 10th Five Year Plan (2002–2007)

In the coming five years, it is proposed that the DMHP will cover 100 districts (about 200 million population). The strength of this approach is the community-based care programme utilizing the primary health care infrastructure. Consequently, the mental health programme budget has been increased from Rs. 28 crores to Rs. 190 crores (a seven-fold increase).

National Health Policy 2002

The National Health Policy (2002) is advocating the organization of a network of decentralized mental health services to tackle common types of disorders:

NHP 2002 envisages a network of decentralized mental health services for ameliorating the more common categories of disorders. The programme outline for such a disease would involve the diagnosis of common disorders, and the prescription of common therapeutic drugs, by general duty medical staff. In regard to mental health institutions for indoor treatment of patients, the Policy envisages the upgrading of the physical infrastructure of such institutions at central government expense so as to secure the human rights of this vulnerable segment of society (p. 32).

Other developments

During the last few years, mental health issues have received attention in a number of other ways. A number of psychiatric centres have been involved in the mental health care of the disaster-affected population (Srinivasa Murthy et al., 1987). This initiative again covers service provision, prevention of mental disorders and promotion of mental health. Efforts to involve families in mental health care have been an ongoing activity in the country since the 1950s. A workshop entitled 'Caring of carers' was organized in May 2001 at Chennai, India. Suicide prevention has been on the agenda (Vijayakumar, 1994), but there are only a dozen suicide prevention initiatives in the whole country. Community care programmes have been developed for the addiction services (Ranganathan, 1996). The Indian Council of Medical Research, New Delhi, is launching a major initiative to research issues in services, generation of new knowledge, monitoring of the community, and research capacity building. Mental health reforms have been initiated in some states (for example, Karnataka and Gujarat).

Agenda for the future

India has developed many innovative approaches to mental health care during the last five decades. The advances in the understanding of human behaviour and mental disorders justify the optimism of developing meaningful and realistic mental health programmes. It is essential to bring the fruits of science to the total population of India. The barriers of lack of awareness of the general population, the occurrence of chronicity and disability, the burden of families providing care, and the lack of institutional infrastructure must be addressed.

The wide variations across the states of India demand that plans are developed for each of the states and union territories, in addition to a national plan and programme. All psychiatric care facilities should be upgraded in terms of trained personnel, treatment and rehabilitation facilities, living arrangements and community outreach activities. All medical colleges should have independent departments of psychiatry to ensure adequate undergraduate training in psychiatry. The current amount of training in psychiatry to medical students needs to be increased. All the districts in India (about 600) should have full mental health teams, as part of district hospitals and the district health office. There should be at least a 10-bed separate psychiatry ward in each district hospital. Integration of mental health with primary health care should be achieved to facilitate early identification of patients, regular treatment and reintegration into the community. The mass media should be utilized fully for public education about mental health and mental disorders. Support from the government for the families of mentally ill people, in terms of community-based services, respite care, help in acute emergencies, financial support, and formation of self-help groups, should be provided.

The full implementation of the Persons with Disabilities Act 1995 and the facilities that are available to the physically handicapped (reservation for employment, social benefits, travel facility, etc.) should be available to people with mental disorders. Special schemes should be set up to support the voluntary agencies to take initiatives towards treatment and rehabilitation of the mentally ill. The involvement of education, labour and welfare in developing mental health programmes is valuable. Planned mental health manpower development by increasing the centres of training and creating opportunities for employment of the trained professionals should be made. Research on issues central to the understanding and treatment of mental disorders should receive support.

Conclusion

India enters the 21st century with many challenges, and developing mental health services is one of these. Progress in implementing mental health programmes has been slow (Srinivasa Murthy and Wig, 1993) but in recent years it has been adequate. Different social institutions have been actively involved in the mental health issues relevant to society. Professionals have been in the forefront of finding solutions appropriate to the country and towards developing an Indian system of mental health care. There are a number of positive developments in the country that have placed mental health in the centre of policy and service development agendas. As happens in any development, there are contrasting forces at work. There are programmes that are not fully developed and there is a need for additional financial, technical and political support. There is also a need for a wider vision for the development of mental health care – one that is broad-based, inclusive of all the needs of all the people, community based and community intensive. Professionals have an important role to guide the development of mental health care in the country.

References

AIR (1995a) Rakesh Chanmd Narayan vs. State of Bihar, SC.208.

AIR (1995b) Supreme Court Legal Aid Committee vs. State of Madhya Pradesh, SC.208.

Amin G, Shah S, Vankar GK (1998) The prevalence and recognition of depression in primary care. Indian Journal of Psychiatry, 40: 364–9.

Bhore J (1946) Health Survey and Development Committee. New Delhi: Government of India.

Bhugra D (2001) The Colonized Psyche: British influence on Indian Psychiatry. In Bhugra D, Littlewood R (Eds.) Colonialism and Psychiatry. Oxford: Oxford University Press.

Central Council of Health and Family Welfare (1982) Ministry of Health and Family Welfare. New Delhi: Government of India.

Central Council of Health and Family Welfare (1999) Ministry of Health and Family Welfare. New Delhi: Government of India.

Chandrasekar CR, Issac MK, Kapur RL, Parthasarathy R (1981) Management of priority mental disorders in the community. Indian Journal of Psychiatry, 23: 174–8.

Channabasavanna SM, Sriram TG, Kishore Kumar K (1995) Results from the Bangalore Centre. In Ustun TB, Sartorius N (Eds.) Mental Illness in General Health Care. Chichester: John Wiley.

Chisholm D, Sekar K, Kishore Kumar K, Saeed K, James S, Mubbashar M, Srinivasa Murthy R (2000) Integration of mental health care into primary health care: Demonstration cost–outcome study in India and Pakistan. British Journal of Psychiatry, 176: 581–8.

Dhanda A (2000) Legal Order, Mental Disorder. New Delhi: Sage.

Frontline (2001) Deliverance in Erwadi. August 18–31.

Frontline (2002) Probe Report on Erwadi. November 22: 132.

Gautam S (1985) Development and evaluation of training programmes for primary mental health care. Indian Journal of Psychiatry, 27: 51–62.

Gautam S, Kapur RL, Shamasundar C (1980) Psychiatric morbidity and referral in General Practice. Indian Journal of Psychiatry, 22: 295–7.

Government of India (2000) Annual Report. Ministry of Health and Family Welfare. New Delhi: Government of India.

Harding TW, de Arango MV, Baltazar J, Climent CE, Ibrahim HHA, Ignacio LL, Srinivasa Murthy R, Wig NN (1980) Mental disorders in primary health care: A study of their frequency and diagnosis in four developing countries. Psychological Medicine, 10: 231–41.

Issac MK, Kapur RL (1980) A cost effectiveness of three different methods of psychiatric case finding in the general population. British Journal of Psychiatry, 137: 540–6.

Issac MK, Kapur RL, Chandrasekar CR, Parthasarathy R, Prema TP (1981) Management of schizophrenics in the community: An experimental report. Indian Journal of Psychological Medicine, 4: 23–7.

Issac MK, Kapur RL, Chandrasekar CR, Kapur M, Parthasarathy R (1982) Mental health delivery in rural primary health care – development and evaluation of a pilot training programme. Indian Journal of Psychiatry, 24: 131–8.

Issac MK, Chandrasekar CR, Parthasarathy R, Srinivasa Murthy R (1986) Decentralised training for PHC medical officers of a district – the Bellary approach. In Verghese A (Ed.) Continuing Medical Education, Vol. VI. Calcutta: Indian Psychiatric Society.

Issac MK, Chandrasekar CR, Srinivasa Murthy R (1988) Manual of mental health care for medical officers. Bangalore: National Institute of Mental Health and Neurosciences.

Manickam LSS (1997) Training community volunteers in preventing alcoholism and drug addiction: A basic programme and its impact on certain variables. Indian Journal of Psychiatry, 39: 220–5.

Menon DK, Manchina M, Dhir A, Srinivasa Murthy R, Wig NN (1978) Training in mental health for community health workers: An experience. In Kumar V (Ed.) Delivery of Health Care in Rural Areas: Chandigarh. PGIMER. pp. 38–41.

Mudaliar AL (1962) Health Survey and Planning Committee. New Delhi: Government of India.

Nagarajiah, Reddamma K, Chandrasekar CR, Issac MK, Srinivasa Murthy R (1994) Evaluation of short-term training in mental health for multipurpose workers. Indian Journal of Psychiatry 36: 12–17.

Naik AN, Isaac M, Parthasarathy R, Karur SV (1994) The perception and experience of health personnel about integration of mental health in general health services. Indian Journal of Psychiatry, 36: 18–21.

Naik AN, Parthasarathy R, Issac MK (1996) Families of rural mentally ill and treatment adherence in district mental health programme. International Journal of Social Psychiatry, 42: 168–72.

National Health Policy (1983) Ministry of Health and Family Welfare. New Delhi: Government of India.

National Health Policy (2002) Ministry of Health and Family Welfare. New Delhi: Government of India.

National Human Rights Commission (1999) Quality Assurance in Mental Health. New Delhi: NHRC.

National Mental Health Programme for India (1982) Ministry of Health and Family Welfare. New Delhi: Government of India.

Parthasarathy R, Chandrasekar CR, Issac MK, Prema TP (1981) A profile of the follow-up of the rural mentally ill. Indian Journal of Psychiatry, 23:139–141.

Patel V (2000) The need for treatment evidence for common mental disorders in developing countries. Psychological Medicine, 30: 743–6.

Patel V, Pereira J, Fernandes J, Mann A (1998) Poverty, psychological disorder and disability in primary care attenders in Goa, India. British Journal of Psychiatry, 172: 533–6.

Pereira J, Patel V (1998) Which antidepressant is best tolerated? A randomised trial of antidepressant treatment for common mental disorders in primary care in Goa. Indian Journal of Psychiatry, 41: 358–63.

Ranganathan S (1996) The empowered community: A paradigm shift in the treatment of alcoholism. Madras: TTR Clinical Research Foundation.

Satyavathi S (1993) Short term training of medical officers in mental health. Indian Journal of Psychiatry, 35: 107–10.

SCC (1982) In Veena Sethi vs. State of Bihar, 2: 583.

Sell HL, Srinivasa Murthy R, Seshadri S, Kumar KVK, Srinivasan K (1989) Recognition and management of patients with functional complaints: A training package for primary health care physicians. New Delhi: WHO Regional Office for South-East Asia.

Sen B (1987) Psychiatric phenomena in primary health care: Their extent and nature. Indian Journal of Psychiatry, 19: 33–40.

Seshadri S, Kumar KVK, Moily S, Srinivasa Murthy R (1988) Patients presenting with multiple somatic complaints to rural health clinic (Sakalawara): Preliminary Report. NIMHANS Journal, 6: 13–17.

Shamasunder C, Kapur RL, Issac MK, Sundaram UK (1983) Orientation course in psychiatry for GPs. Indian Journal of Psychiatry, 25: 288–90.

Shamasunder C, Kapur RL, Sundaram UK, Pai S, Nagarathna GN (1986) Involvement of the GPs in urban mental health care. Journal of Indian Medical Association, 72: 310–13.

Sharma SD (1986) Psychiatry in primary care. Ranchi: Central Institute of Psychiatry.

Shaw WS (1932) The alienist department of India. Journal of Mental Science, 78: 331–41.

Somasundaram O (1973) Religious treatment in Tamil Nadu. Indian Journal of Psychiatry, 15: 38–42.

Srinivasa Murthy R, Wig NN (1993) Evaluation of the progress in mental health in India since independence. In Mane P and Gandevia K (Eds.) Mental health in India. Tata Institute of Social Sciences. pp. 387–405.

Srinivasa Murthy R, Wig NN (2002) Psychiatric diagnosis and classification in developing countries. In Maj M, Lopez Ibor W, Sartorus N (Eds.) Psychiatric Diagnosis and Classification. London: Wiley. pp. 249–79.

Srinivasa Murthy R, Ghosh A, Wig NN (1974) Treatment acceptance patterns in a psychiatric out-patient clinic – study of demographic and clinical variables. Indian Journal of Psychiatry, 16: 323–30.

Srinivasa Murthy R, Kuruvilla K, Verghese A, Pulimood BM (1976) Psychiatric illness in a general hospital clinic. Journal of Indian Medical Association, 66: 6–8.

Srinivasa Murthy R, Chandrasekar CR, Nagarajiah, Issac MK, Parthasathy R, Raghuram A (1988) Manual of mental health care for multi-purpose workers. Bangalore: National Institute of Mental Health and Neurosciences.

Srinivasa Murthy R, Kaur R, Wig NN (1978) Mentally ill in a rural community: Some initial experiences in case identification and management. Indian Journal of Psychiatry, 20: 143–7.

Srinivasa Murthy R, Issac MK, Chandrasekar CR, Bhide A (1987) Manual of mental health for medical officers – Bhopal disaster. New Delhi: Indian Council of Medical Research.

Sriram TG, Kishore K, Moily S, Chandrasekar CR, Issac MK, Srinivasa Murthy R, (1987) Minor psychiatric disturbances in primary health care: A study of their prevalence and characteristics using a simple case detection technique. Indian Journal of Social Psychiatry, 3: 212–26.

Sriram TG, Chandrasekar CR, Moily S, Kumar K, Raghuram A, Issac MK, Srinivasa Murthy R (1989) Standardisation of multiple-choice questionnaire for evaluation medical officers training in psychiatry. Social Psychiatry and Psychiatric Epidemiology, 24: 327–31.

Sriram TG, Moily S, Kumar GS, Chandrasekar CR, Issac MK, Srinivasa Murthy R (1990a) Training of primary health care medical officers in mental health care. Errors in clinical judgement before and after training. General Hospital Psychiatry, 12: 384–9.

Sriram TG, Chandrasekar CR, Issac MK, Srinivasa Murthy R, Moily S, Kumar K, Shanmugam V (1990b) Development of case vignettes to assess the mental health training of primary care medical officers. Acta Psychiatrica Scandinavica, 82: 174–7.

Sriram TG, Chandrasekar CR, Issac MK, Srinivasa Murthy R, Shanmugam V (1990c) Training primary care medical officers in mental health care: An evaluation using multiple-choice questionnaire. Acta Psychiatrica Scandinavica, 81: 414–17.

Sriram TG, Srinivasa Murthy R, Issac MK, Chandrasekar CR (1991) Manual of psychotherapy for medical officers. Bangalore: National Institute of Mental Health and Neurosciences.

Supreme Court Commission Report (1984) Enquiry report on Hospital for Mental Diseases. Delhi: Shahadra.

Varma LP (1953) History of psychiatry in India and Pakistan. Journal of Neurology and Psychiatry, 4: 26–8.

Vijayakumar L (1994) Befriending the suicidal in India. Crisis, 15: 99–100.

Wig NN (1978) General hospital psychiatry units – a right time for evaluation. Indian Journal of Psychiatry, 20: 1–5.

Wig NN, Parhee R (1984) Manual of mental disorders for primary health care physicians. New Delhi: Indian Council of Medical Research.

Wig NN, Srinivasa Murthy R (1980) Manual of mental disorders for peripheral health personnel. Published by Department of Psychiatry. PGIMER Chandigarh (2nd printing 1993).

Wig NN, Srinivasa Murthy R (1981a) Reaching the unreached – II. Experiments in organising rural psychiatric services. Indian Journal of Psychological Medicine, 4: 47–52.

Wig NN, Srinivasa Murthy R, Harding TW (1981b) A model for rural psychiatric services – Raipur Rani experience. Indian Journal of Psychiatry, 23: 275–90.

Wig NN, Srinivasa Murthy R, Manchina M, Arpan D (1980) Psychiatric services through peripheral health centres. Indian Journal of Psychiatry, 22: 311–16.

CHAPTER SEVEN

Mental health policy in Brazil: From dictatorship to democracy

WILLIANS VALENTINI AND DOMINGOS NASCIMENTO ALVES

Introduction

Brazil is a federated republic composed of 26 states, a Federal District, and more than 5000 municipalities. The public health sector, called the Unified Public Health System [*Sistema Único de Saúde*], or SUS, is universal, and operates in conjunction with private systems, consisting of health care and health insurance companies. More than 60% of the Brazilian population is treated exclusively by the public system.

The Unified Public Health System was instituted by the Federal Constitution of 1988, which marked the end of the country's last period of dictatorship. The system is regulated by Laws 8.080 and 8.142, of December 1990, which determine:

- The universal right to health and health care in a just and integral manner.
- Unified organization, under the responsibility of the three levels of government – federal, state and municipal.
- Social control, exercised by various actors, such as associations of health professionals, families and users, as well as other representative segments of Brazilian society.

The social participation in formulating and following up on health policies is regulated by the aforementioned Law 8.142, which provides that such participation should take the form of representation in collective organs, specifically, health boards and health conferences. The latter are held in municipal, state and national stages.

From the legal standpoint, the system is broad and democratic. It therefore represents an enormous step forward in the establishment of social rights, in comparison with the previous system, which served only the beneficiaries of governmental social security institutes.

The major historical events on the road to reforming psychiatric treatment and mental health policies over the last 15 years can be summarized chronologically as follows:

- First National Mental Health Conference – 1987.
- National Congress of the Mental Health Workers' Movement, Bauru – 1987.
- Intervention in the Anchieta Hospital, Santos – 1989.
- Presentation in the Federal Chamber of Deputies of a bill presented by Deputy Paulo Delgado, in 1989.
- Declaration of Caracas, 1990.
- Publication of the first rulings, to support financially the change in the model of treatment, was made by the Health Ministry in 1991; the most recent law dealing with this question is No. 10.216, of 6 April 2001.

Basically this last law defines the progressive substitution of the hospital model with the open community services model. It also allows a legally instituted authority to question involuntary admission to a mental hospital and lists a number of rights of persons with mental disorders when submitted to any treatment. In addition, the excessive length of time required for this law to be passed led state and municipal legislators to approve other laws on their respective levels, also based on the original bill of 1989.

Historical background

As is true in almost all Western countries, the history of psychiatry in Brazil begins with the opening of its first psychiatric hospital. The Pedro II Asylum, named after the then Emperor of Brazil, was opened in 1852 in Rio de Janeiro, capital of the empire. This asylum was subordinated to the Santa Casa general hospital, directed by a Roman Catholic institution. Treatment was typical of the times, consisting of moral postures and strict discipline (Costa, 1981).

Pedro II Asylum entered a period of crisis even before the fall of the empire, in 1889, as the number of patients exceeded the institution's capacity. The attending physicians took over direction of its management and before the end of the 19th century, began setting up 'Colonies of Alienated Persons', which were large hospitals located on the outskirts of important cities. The first of such institutions in Latin America were the São Bento and the Conde de Mesquita asylums, on Ilha do Governador, near Rio de Janeiro (Amarante, 1994).

Many other such institutions were established in other states around the country shortly after the proclamation of the Republic in 1889, and this type of approach dominated psychiatric treatment during the entire first half of the 20th century. Unfortunately, almost all became infamous, such as that at Juqueri, near São Paulo, and at Juliano Moreira, in Rio de Janeiro.

Psychiatry was legitimated at the beginning of the Republic, with the promulgation of a specific law that organized assistance to the 'alienated'. The Brazilian Mental Hygiene League was created in 1923, whose charter of principles set down 'a programme of intervention in social space, with markedly eugenistic, xenophobic, anti-liberal and racist characteristics' (Amarante, 1994).

Psychiatry, with its exceptional instrument of intervention, the asylum, was of course organized for the poor. The practices carried out at the asylums continued to consist of moral treatment until the 1930s, with the appearance of 'new' practices, then under the influence of German psychiatry. These practices included electroconvulsive therapy, insulin or cardiazolic shocks, and lobotomies (Amarante, 1994).

In the 1960s, the country was under a full-blown military dictatorship, and intense industrialization was taking place, associated with migration of the rural population to the large cities and the expansion of the middle class, a segment that had historically enjoyed a certain amount of public social security. The model of large colonies for the mentally ill, already in decline, was progressively replaced by private psychiatric hospitals, contracted by the National Social Security Institute, which was set up in Brazil through an authoritarian process of unification of the former variety of social security institutes, mentioned above (Oliveira and Teixeira, 1986).

This period, which became known in psychiatric circles as the times of the 'industry of madness', saw an absurd growth in the number of private beds contracted for mental patients (Cerqueira, 1984).

In the late 1970s, the military dictatorship was facing problems of legitimacy resulting from the economic recession in the country and from other factors, including the increasing dissension within the political forces that had until then sustained the regime. The National Social Security System also entered into a severe financial crisis.

An important variable that favoured public discussion of psychiatric treatment was the end of the censorship of the press in 1979. This fact allowed the appearance of countless accusations of mistreatment in mental hospitals around the country, which brought the appalling situation of traditional psychiatric treatment to public attention. Franco Basaglia, visiting a psychiatric hospital in the city of Barbacena, Minas Gerais, in 1979, called it a 'public gaolhouse' and referred to the psychiatrists as 'prison wardens' (Firmino, 1982).

There has been increasing discussion about the miserable living conditions under which thousands of mental patients around the world have lived, especially since the end of World War II. The 1960s and 1970s benefited from contributions from Erving Goffman, especially after the publication of his book *Asylums* (Goffman, 1961). Goffman's thinking influenced the generation of professionals of the 1960s and 1970s, and is now also influencing the generation of those who graduated during the 1990s. Disclosures of the execution by the Nazis of more than one million mental patients in Germany between 1933 and 1945 (Muller Hill, 1989) also helped strengthen the struggle in favour of respect for human rights worldwide.

In 1975, at the high point of the repression imposed by the military regime in Brazil, Michel Foucault spent some time at the University of São Paulo, giving seminars which continue to inspire directions for implementing new forms of psychiatric care. Another major influence in the process of psychiatric reform in Brazil is related to experiences in Italy, mainly in Trieste, and the consequences of the approval of Law 180 in that country.

With the end of the military dictatorship in Brazil, the state governors were freely elected in late 1982. A process of change soon began in the field of mental health, contrary to the logic of giving privilege to psychiatric hospitals. In some states funds then began to be channelled to the founding of out-patient mental health clinics. This process culminated in at least a moderate reduction in the number of psychiatric hospital admissions, a fact which contributed to the interruption in the exponential growth in the number of mental asylums in the country.

In São Paulo, in 1983, seven imprisoned mental health patients who had tried to escape from the mental hospital/prison at Franco da Rocha, near São Paulo, were murdered by the military police. In this first year of democratic state governments, which had been elected after the end of the dictatorship, the gravity of this execution resulted in mobilization of the public and the founding of the Teotônio Vilela Human Rights Committee. This committee is composed of Brazilian citizens of high respectability and national visibility, including a federal senator, a federal deputy, a state deputy, and intellectuals committed to the struggle for respect for human rights.

This committee still functions today, promoting respect for Brazilian and international human rights conventions. Its purpose is to follow up on and publicize cases of mass murders and atrocities committed against defenceless citizens who are hospitalized or imprisoned, including the determination of responsibilities. The visibility of the committee's work has contributed greatly to strengthen criticisms regarding the conditions of hospitalization of persons with mental disorders in Brazilian mental asylums.

The resumption of the democratic process, which began in 1982, made the year of 1983 fertile in other initiatives related to the struggle for the expansion of freedom and greater commitment to citizens' rights. The Sixth International and Third National Congresses of the Network for Alternatives to Psychiatry were held in Belo Horizonte in 1983. Many of the measures designed to defend the human rights of Brazilian mental patients in place today were first promoted during those meetings.

In the city of São Paulo, also in 1983, the local group of militants from the Network of Alternatives to Psychiatry organized the 'Franco Basaglia tribunal' at one of the city's cultural centres. More than 1,000 people took part in this event, at which accusations of violent treatment were presented. The tribunal was publicized in the national press and televised media.

This fact, among others, increased coverage in the media of accusations of inhumane treatment and violation of rights in psychiatric hospitals. At the beginning, the appalling conditions of the functioning of asylums were exposed, especially of public psychiatric hospitals managed by state governments.

The First National Conference on Mental Health was held in Rio de Janeiro in 1987. One thousand mental health professionals were present at this event, but very few service users. The need for changes in the psychiatric treatment model in Brazil was endorsed, based almost exclusively on the extremely low quality of the hospital care afforded. The basic rights of the patients in these institutions were frequently violated, and the impermeability of the institutions to social reform became clear. Such services nevertheless exerted strong pressure on the state governments, since 80% of the hospital system consisted of private services contracted by the state. This first conference therefore had the merit of establishing a minimum consensus around the need to restructure the care afforded.

At the Second Congress of Mental Health Workers, also held in 1987, in the city of Bauru, SP, the subject under discussion was 'For a society without mental asylums'. After several years this motto became the theme for the foundation of the National Anti-Asylum Movement, which has exercised a very positive influence on the formulation of public policies regarding mental health in almost all the states in the country, besides having been an important instrument for informing public opinion and prompting legislators to pass favourable federal and state laws.

Finally, also in 1987, the first Psychosocial Treatment Centre [*Centros de Atenção Psicossocial*], or CAPS, was founded in the country's largest city, São Paulo. This centre eventually became a model for what later evolved into what is now known as 'the expanded clinic', consisting of full treatment for persons with serious mental disorders, provided in day-hospital regimes and operated by a multidisciplinary team. Services funded by community and social resources are rendered. The plan also includes an intensive support programme for relatives of the users of the services.

Contemporary profile

The Federative Republic of Brazil is the largest country in South America, with 170 million inhabitants. It has the world's ninth largest economy, with a GNP of approximately US$750 billion and yearly per capita income of approximately US$3,500. It is one of the most unjust countries in the world, being listed in 73rd place on the Human Development Index (2001) (United Nations Development Program, 2002) with an extremely imbalanced income distribution in favour of an oligarchy which controls the financial system and some industrial sectors (United Nations Development Program, 2002).

Another basic characteristic of the country's instability is the existence of vast land-holdings. It has not yet been possible to implement any land reform and there remain enormous areas of land in the hands of a very few owners. The political confrontation against this imbalance is being led mainly by the Landless Rural Workers' Movement, a grassroots organization composed of Brazilian peasants who struggle for the ownership of land on which to settle and produce food.

Brazil also has great regional inequalities. The southern and southeastern regions of the country concentrate the greatest wealth, whereas the northeast shows the lowest rates of social development. The economy is based on a diversified industrial production, on farming and, in some cities and in the northeast, on tourism, a sector that favours regional economies.

The ethnic composition of the population shows great regional variations. In the northern and central-western regions, white European descendants and mestizos (Caucasian with native Brazilian) predominate. In the northeast and southeast, there is considerable miscegenation of Caucasians with Afro-Brazilians, resulting in a large mixed-race population. The south was more strongly influenced by intense European immigration during the last two centuries, and therefore has a predominantly Caucasian population. Literacy rates are low, even by Latin-American standards, with about 87% of the population having only minimum educational levels.

The Unified Public Health System (SUS), established by law in 1990, is in a process of consolidation, with progressive transfer of responsibilities and funds to the municipal level. This process is currently hampered by the federal fiscal adjustment policy that has been in effect over the last few years, within a political and administrative context which tends towards the recentralization of financial resources. Per capita expenditure on health is currently around US$100 per year.

In the field of Latin-American mental health policies, the Pan-American Health Organization (PAHO) held the Regional Conference for Restructuring Psychiatric Care in South America, in Caracas, Venezuela, in

November of 1990. The conference produced the 'Declaration of Caracas', which basically proposed:

• Phasing out of psychiatric hospitals as the central service offered in the area of mental health.
• Humanization of psychiatric hospitals.
• Broadening of the rights of persons with mental disorders.

The Declaration of Caracas had significant repercussions across the South-American continent, especially in Brazil. As we shall see, in recent years the principles contained in it have helped sustain strategies for restructuring mental health care and have served as a reference document for related policies.

After the announcement of new perspectives and changes to be implemented throughout Latin America, begun by the Declaration, a workshop sponsored by the PAHO/WHO was held in the city of Santos, by the Health Ministry and the Municipal Government, in June 1991. This workshop was one of the first measures in the preparation of the Second National Mental Health Conference.

The first step was to invite the then 12 Brazilian associations of users and families to a meeting sponsored by the Health Ministry and the São Paulo Municipal Government, in December of the same year, with the objectives of encouraging them to publicize their activities and actions and elect their representatives to the conference's organizing committee.

The process of holding the Second National Conference resulted from the mobilization of over 20,000 people nationwide. More than 100 municipal conferences and 24 state conferences were held. The national phase, held in Brasilia in December, 1992, had over 1,000 participants, including voting delegates, participants, and guests from other countries. Approximately 100 users of mental health services and about the same number of family members also took part in this last stage (Brasil, 1994).

The active participation of many users and family members in all stages showed their interest and effectiveness in defining policies in this field. It also evidenced a very specific characteristic of Brazilian associations, which are usually mixed, placing health professionals side by side with users and family members. These groups are almost always associated with some specific mental health care institution (Fernandes, 1996).

A determining issue, which occurred two years before the Second Conference, was the presentation in the Federal Chamber of Deputies of a bill drawn up by Deputy Paulo Delgado, regulating the 'progressive phasing out of psychiatric hospitals in Brazil'. Considerable debate ensued, but the bill remained 'in hospital' in the National Congress for 12 years. It was submitted to all kinds of pressure, especially from groups representing corporate and financial interests.

The long period this bill took to move through Congress gives a clear idea of the difficulties faced in this country in regard to the dominant mentality that promotes exclusion and supports specific interests. However, the drawing up and approving of public policies is no more than a part of the challenges to be overcome for consolidating the new proposed model.

At the same time, in line with the social debate and backed up by the Declaration of Caracas, the Health Ministry took the following decisions as of 1991:

- To change the system for financing mental health provision in the Table of Procedures of the Unified Health System.
- To set up a permanent collegiate board of state mental health co-ordinators/consultants to co-ordinate the process of change.
- To maintain channels of communication and support with public opinion by summoning the Second National Mental Health Conference.
- To advise Congress in order to change current psychiatric legislation.
- To provide more international interchange with consultation from the PAHO/WHO (Alves, 1996).

At this time, a multicentre study on psychiatric morbidity held in the largest cities of three different states showed a potential demand for psychiatric care varying from 19% to 34%. Alcohol abuse and dependence appeared at the time as the most serious problem, affecting between 11% and 15% of the male population. Alcoholic psychosis and abstinence syndrome represented the second and fourth causes, respectively, of psychiatric hospital admissions in the public system in 1992 (Datasus, 1992).

Some results of the process of restructuring mental health care in Brazil are outlined in the Tables 7.1 and 7.2.

In spite of the 30% fall in the number of beds in psychiatric hospitals, there is no lack of psychiatric care, because the hospitals are being replaced by community services, called, in this report, Psychosocial Care Centres (CAPS/NAPS).

Table 7.3 shows the evolution of the number of substitute services in Brazil between 1997 and 2002.

Also in the field of governmental policies on the three levels of the SUS Public Health System, we would call attention to the publication in 2000 of Ruling 106, which regulates the functioning of protective homes for the mentally ill, herein called 'residential therapeutic services'. These institutions are a powerful instrument for replacing the questionable 'hospitality' of mental asylums. The states of Rio de Janeiro and Minas Gerais have provisions in place to transfer financial resources from psychiatric hospitals to the services mentioned above.

Table 7.1 Reduction in the number of psychiatric hospitals 1991–2001

	1991	1996	2001
Public	54	50	50
Contracted	259	219	210
Total	313	269	260

Source: Ministry of Health, 2001

Table 7.2 Reduction in the number of psychiatric hospital beds 1991–2001

	1991	1996	2001
Public	19,551	14,902	11,697
Contracted	65,486	53,560	40,889
Total	85,037	67,462	52,586

Source: Ministry of Health, 2001

Table 7.3 Evolution of CAPS/NAPS (treatment centres) in the SUS system 1997–2002

1997	1998	1999	2001	2002
176	231	237	295	382

Source: Information Bulletin, Number 3, Ministry of Health, 2002

In the field of social mobilization, two important facts stand out: the holding of the Second National Congress of Users and Family Members, in the city of Santos, in December, 1993, where the 'Charter of Rights of Users in Brazil' was approved; and the holding of five National Encounters of the Movement Against Asylums, in 1993 and 2001. Each of these events had over 500 participants, including users, family members, and health professionals.

Despite the unmistakable inroads made in recent years, some difficulties still need to be overcome, especially the strong concentration of funds in the sphere of the hospitals, currently representing 90% of expenditure on psychiatric care. This fact evidences an unquestionable contradiction between the accumulated experience of recent decades, and the allocation of resources. Besides being relatively recent, the instruments for reallocating resources are scattered among the three levels of the public system. They are based on a model of defraying costs for activities that are largely centralized at the federal level. The process of decentralization is chaotic and is occurring in a period of recessive fiscal policies and with a strong tendency towards centralization.

Another challenge to be faced is the formation and training of health professionals to work under the new model. The hegemonic standard of medical education in Brazil is based on the model formulated by Flexner during the 1950s, featuring high specialization, with great importance given to nosological aspects in detriment to other determinants of illness, and hierarchical and backward clinical practice. However, there is a current trend towards reversing this hegemony, even though the former model is defended in university circles, exactly where changes should be fostered.

Brazil's public universities, but even more so its non-public universities, are basically geared towards the formation and training of professionals for the private labour market. There is little or no concern for models concerned with collective health, which are usually considered 'problems for the government to handle', while in practice the universities train armies of practitioners with questionable clinical protocols and uncritical postures regarding the exercise of their profession. Such groups also defend social control through very strong corporate organizations, and react against the democratization of the exercise of their profession.

The lacuna in the training for contemporary practices that are compatible with more recent ethical and technical presuppositions is being filled in with what is referred to here as an 'expanded clinic'. This scheme is composed of training programmes in community services. Some universities have included this form of work in their curricula with encouragement from departments that accept the new model.

The difficulty in finding well-trained professionals, especially physicians, for practices that take into account 'the problem', and not merely the diagnosis, is aggravated by the still predominant prerogative of psychiatrists to hospitalize – with the complicity of other professional categories – without adequate justification, as this has only recently been required, with the passage of the new law. The Brazilian situation bears the weight of over 200 years of unfortunate practices that must be reviewed and overcome if the older model is to be replaced by a democratized system.

The implementation of psychiatric reform in Brazil is moving ahead, within lines of action based on the development of the country's democratic process. Health boards, educational boards, and social service boards are thus being implemented at municipal, state and national levels.

It should be noted that the work and thinking of Franco Basaglia, Franca Ongaro Basaglia, Franco Rotelli, and other protagonists of the process of replacing mental asylums in Italy continue to influence Brazilian psychiatric reform. In addition, during all of the 1990s this reform has been influenced by the more recent ideas of Benedetto Saraceno, especially with respect to the development of processes for the psychosocial rehabilitation of patients (Saraceno, 2001).

The participation of patients and their families, as well as of professional associations, has changed the passive behaviour of society towards ineffective or questionable measures that have traditionally been taken regarding persons with mental disorders. This sector of society is already weighed down with disadvantages, including the fact that such persons are usually poor, therefore marginalized from the social process in general and excluded from their condition as citizens by legislation from the fascist period of 1934, which has only recently been partially revoked.

Despite the perspectives for the success of the new mental health policy, especially after the enactment of Law 10.216, there is still much to do. Deplorable scenes were observed in several of the 20 psychiatric hospitals visited in the year 2000 by the Human Rights Committee of the Federal Chamber of Deputies, known as the 'Caravan for Citizenship'. It became clear that broad transformations in the everyday life of people and in their places of residence still need to take place if a better future is to be guaranteed for mental patients who receive specialized treatment.

In this process of democratization, citizens who represent the various groups participate and then often become members of the boards described above, with defined terms of office and responsibilities. In turn, participating in such activities gives the representatives an opportunity to learn more about the complex process of transferring to the municipalities the managerial and executive responsibility over policies, since these have historically been centralized by the federal government.

Only by strengthening citizenship and the democratic process of participation has it been possible to expose the inner workings of institutions that violate human rights. Many private profit-making psychiatric hospitals have been closed down by the government. In addition, many of the institutions that violated human rights and abused their power to hospitalize saw their contracts with the public authority rescinded, and consequently also closed their doors.

The Third National Mental Health Conference was held in December, 2001, with the theme of 'Dare to Care! Stop Exclusion!' – a motto coined by the World Health Organization for the worldwide Mental Health Day celebrated in the year 2001. This was a highly successful event, especially since it was preceded by 115 municipal and/or regional conferences and 27 state conferences. Later, 1,480 people participated in the subsequent national conference, among whom were 11 foreign guests (Brasil – Ministério da Saúde, 2002). The conference strengthened the restructuring process now under way and served as a powerful demonstration of the political strength of the agents involved in the reform. This was demonstrated by the fact that no recommendation considered incompatible with the new law was approved.

The process of reform in Brazil has had very definite effects, since no community service opened in the last 10 years has had to close, nor have any new psychiatric hospitals begun operating. However, the pace of the changes varies greatly from one region of the country to another. Nevertheless, more than five years after the restructuring of psychiatric care, successful experiences can be reported in all of the regions except the northern region, where there are an insignificant number of mental hospitals.

Case studies

A number of investigations have been carried out in the southeastern region of Brazil, which has the country's highest gross product.

In 1989 – one year after the promulgation of the 1988 Federal Constitution, often referred to as the Citizens' Constitution – the city of Santos, state of São Paulo, took an unprecedented measure in the history of Brazilian psychiatry. This beach and port city, having a population of over 400,000 people and located 70 km from São Paulo, had a highly profitable private psychiatric hospital authorized for 260 patients. In fact, it was housing 575 mental patients, many of them hospitalized for alcoholism.

Numerous accusations of mistreatment and death through violence led the state government to carry out an evaluation of the hospital, which took place in March of 1989 but resulted in no sanction against the psychiatrist owners. The Municipal Secretary of Health at the time, David Capistrano da Costa Filho, with the evaluation report in hand and using the powers vested in him by the Federal Constitution, initiated a process of intervention in the psychiatric hospital and dismissed not only the hospital's owners, but also its contracted physicians and other university-trained professionals, all of whom were considered co-responsible for the violence against the patients.

Since this intervention, five mental health centres, called Psychosocial Attention Centres (NAPS) have been implemented, similar to the model used in Trieste. With the participation of users' associations and public functionaries, this chain of centres evolved to the point that workshops were set up to provide the patients with paid work. The psychiatric hospital was eventually shut down. This experience is still one of the most important examples of the process of change going on in the country.

In 1990, under the influence of the experience in Santos, which had indicated a possible direction for dealing with psychiatric professionals guilty of violating patients' human rights, a different situation arose in the city of Campinas, also in southeastern Brazil, located 90 km north of São Paulo, with a population of 800,000 inhabitants. There the municipal government signed a co-management contract with a philanthropic mental asylum – Dr Cândido Ferreira Sanatorium – as this institution was undergoing administrative and financial difficulties.

At the time, Campinas had over 1,200 psychiatric beds in five private profit-making psychiatric hospitals. The process of change in the model of care under way since then has been proof of the feasibility of the recommendations contained in the Declaration of Caracas, as well as of the basic principles of the Unified Health System, Human Rights Conventions, and the Brazilian Psychiatric Reform.

With a total of 194 resident patients and a staff of 60 at that time, the institution's care practices began to undergo revision. Interaction with the community was initiated, and treatment was also made available in the downtown area. Today over 300 health professionals work with over 1,000 patients, treated via a system of individual therapeutic projects. There are also 25 houses which lodge 130 former hospitalized patients in various neighbourhoods in the city. Ten workshops employ and pay over 230 clients, organized into labour co-operatives. All these clients now use the income they receive from their work to contribute to their family incomes or to defray the expenses of the homes where they live.

During the years 2001 and 2002 the partnership between Candido Ferreira and the municipal government was responsible for the creation of four new Psychosocial Treatment Centres (CAPS) in four different health districts, in the urban area of the city. All the centres are open 24 hours a day, seven days a week, and also offer care for acute patients. The new centres employed mental health workers from the last private psychiatric hospital to close in 2001. The partnership is also responsible for the presence of more than 500 community health agents who are responsible for the health of the population that live in all the peripheral areas of the city.

Since 1991, the town of Angra dos Reis, a beach city in the State of Rio de Janeiro of approximately 95,000 inhabitants, has been restructuring its mental health service. Its system is now based on a Psychosocial Treatment Centre (CAPS), including psychiatric beds in the general hospital and a prize-winning and creative programme called 'Back Home'. The city government set up a house for each municipal citizen who had had hospitalized in a psychiatric hospital for a long period. Former patients who found it difficult to return to their original families had the option of having a relative live with them (Pitta, 1996).

The city of Rio de Janeiro was the scene of another positive experience. Rio had been the capital of the Empire and the Republic of Brazil until 1960. By then a large number of beds existed in public and contracted private psychiatric hospitals, making it the city with the highest number of beds in the country. Since the 1980s, measures have been taken to humanize the public hospitals which, during that decade, played a major role as a vanguard sector.

More recently, as of the mid-1990s, the municipality has established consistent guidelines for restructuring the care provided. This has included control over the number of hospital admissions, reduction in the number of contracted beds, and implementation of a network of Psychosocial

Treatment Centres in the poorest areas in the city. To date, 11 homes have been opened.

The results are visible: more than 2,000 beds were deactivated in five years, and there has been strong social legitimization of the community work and pioneer initiatives, such as legislation to grant a monthly allowance to families of patients who have been hospitalized in psychiatric hospitals for more than three years.

There are still 3,500 beds in existence, 1,300 of which are public, in a city of almost 6 million inhabitants. A high percentage of Rio's population still lives below the poverty line, but, despite this, the city has shown that it can do away with mental asylums.

Proof of this statement is the stimulating project known as 'Back to Citizenship'. This programme provides care to children and adolescents with serious mental deficiencies who were formerly hospitalized in shelters for minors, and later absorbed by their families. The city guarantees proper and regular care, and financial support of approximately U$350 per month. Some of the children have been placed in monitored homes, with integration into the life of the city (Delgado and Almeida, 2000).

Betim, in the state of Minas Gerais, is an industrial city of 300,000 inhabitants, located near the state capital of Belo Horizonte. Approximately 100 persons with mental disorders were traditionally sent per month to psychiatric hospitals in Belo Horizonte. In the early 1990s a process of reform was begun.

The city set up a Psychosocial Treatment Centre for adults, open 24 hours a day, and another for children and adolescents. It also kept strict control over the hospitalization of its citizens, which has become a rare event: fewer than 10 per year, for the last five years. The success of the process in Betim influenced many other municipalities, due to the effectiveness of the programme and its widespread social acceptance and approval.

The northeastern region of Brazil presents the worst indicators of human development. Natal, the coastal capital city of the state of Rio Grande do Norte, with approximately 800,000 inhabitants, has a public psychiatric hospital and two private hospitals, contracted by the city, with a total of 534 beds.

In 1994, when the restructuring process began and the first Psychosocial Care Centres were opened, the city had 764 beds. Today the mental health programme consists of two such centres, one especially for clientele with problems related to alcohol and drug abuse. Other professionals associated with the programme work in 60 basic health units and participate in the Family Health Programme by supervising its teams. The system also includes five beds at the general hospital of the public university. In 2000 the Locomotive Project was launched, consisting of a labour co-operative

which, besides producing items for sale, has become an important instrument for publicizing the principles of the reform to local society.

Also in the northeast, the city of Quixadá, with 60,000 inhabitants, located in the backlands of the state of Ceará, used to send approximately 100
mental patients per year for admission to psychiatric hospitals located 200
km away, in the state capital of Fortaleza. Since 1993, with the implementation of a Psychosocial Treatment Centre, the number of persons
admitted to psychiatric hospitals was reduced to four per year. Psychiatric
crises are treated by admission to the city's general hospital, and follow-up
is carried out through care projects, with responsibility shared with the
families.

Several thousand kilometres away, the southern region of the country
presents the highest human development indicators. The city of São
Lourenço do Sul, in the state of Rio Grande do Sul, has a community
service programme also worthy of mention, called 'Our House'. This institution is responsible for treating people suffering from mental disorders,
with responsibilities being shared among the multiprofessional team
members, patients, families, neighbours, and volunteers.

Also in the state of Rio Grande do Sul, the city of Bagé, with approximately 120,000 inhabitants, organized a Community Mental Health
Service in the early 1990s. The professionals of that city have exerted great
efforts to modify the population's image of madness, and have been successful in obtaining considerable social approval for the theme of
psychiatric reform. The city opened up its first shelter in the mid-1990s,
providing a home for 10 former in-patients of a local psychiatric hospital.

Summary

In Brazil, during the last 20 years, several important changes have occurred
in psychiatric assistance. The most important changes began with the
process of humanization of psychiatric assistance initiated in the 1980s,
after the end of the military period. A community mental health model is
now in the process of implementation.

The most important axes for the transformation of the model are the
Psychosocial Treatment Centres and the Family Health Programme, which
includes the work of the Community Health Agents, covering most of the
national territory.

These changes are taking place at the same time as broad socio-political
changes for the re-democratization of the country and also for the development of the SUS (Unified Public Health System). The process is being
conducted under the orientation of social participation, involving health
councils in all the governmental spheres and municipal, state and national

conferences. The future has been announced, the main trends have been defined, and the substitution of the old model for a community one is progressing.

References

Alves DS (1996) Reestruturación de los Servicios de Salud Mental en Brasil. Psiquiatria Pública, 8 (4). Madrid.

Amarante P (1994) Psiquiatria Social e Reforma Psiquiátrica. Rio de Janeiro: Editora Fiocruz.

Datasus (1992) Data Bank of the Ministry of Health, Brazil.

Brasil-Ministério da Saúde (1994) Relatório Final da 2ª Conferência Nacional de Saúde Mental. Coordinação de Saúde Mental/MS, Brasília.

Brasil-Ministério da Saúde (2002) Conselho Nacional de Saúde. Relatório Final da III Conferência Nacional de Saúde Mental/MS, Brasília.

Cerqueira L (1984) Psiquiatria Social: Problemas Brasileiros de Saúde Mental. Rio de Janeiro and São Paulo: Livraria Atheneu.

Costa JF (1981) História da Psiquiatria no Brasil. Rio de Janeiro: Editora Campus.

Delgado PG, Almeida NC (2000) De Volta à cidadania: Políticas públicas para crianças e adolescentes. Rio de Janeiro: Editora Té Corá e Instituto Franco Basaglia.

Fernandes G (1996) Organizacion Panamericana de la Salud. Reunión de Evaluación de la Iniciativa para la Reestruturación de la Atención Psiquiátrica en América Latina. Panamá: Mimeo.

Firmino H (1982) Nos Porões da Loucura. Rio de Janeiro: Editora Codecri.

Goffman E (1961) Asylums. Harmondsworth: Penguin.

Ministry of Health (2001) Mental Health Technical Advisorship Report, Health Assistant Secretary. Ministry of Health, Brazil.

Ministry of Health (2002) Information Bulletin Number 3, Mental Health Technical Advisorship, Health Assistant Secretary. Ministry of Health, Brazil.

Muller Hill B (1989) Scienza di Morte. L'eliminazione degli ebrei, degli zigani e malati di mente. 1933–1945. Milan, Italy: ETS.

Oliveira JA, Teixeira SF (1986) Previdência Social: 60 anos de história da Previdência no Brasil. Petrópolis/RJ: Vozes.

Pitta A (1996) Reabilitação Psicossocial no Brasil. São Paulo: Editora HUCITEC.

Saraceno B (2001) Libertando Identidades: Da reabilitação psicosocial à cidadania possível. Rio de Janeiro: Editora Té Corá e Instituto Franco Basaglia.

United Nations Development Program (2002) Human Development Report 2002. New York: Oxford University Press.

YURI S. SAVENKO

CHAPTER EIGHT
Russia: Mental health reform in the post-Soviet period

Introduction

The main driving force for the care of the mental health of a population and the efforts for organization of psychiatric care are a natural practical need. The forms which these efforts require reflect both the condition of society itself, and the direction taken for social development. As a result, the status of psychiatric practice is one of the most subtle indicators of the social dynamics and tendencies taking shape within a nation.

An analysis of the problem of prophylaxis in the history of Russian psychiatry, in the context of sociopolitical and cultural development, affirms that mindsets and practices pertaining to the mental health of the population arise out of the structure of society itself. Various social systems, with differing priorities, settle this problem in different ways. Totalitarian and authoritarian systems give priority to state and empire; traditional and theocratic systems emphasize the priority of society; democratic systems give priority to the individual. The psychiatric service in each system may be evaluated from the point of view of its own 'realities' and criteria, and from the positions of the other two social systems.

The problem of mental health policy is first of all a sociological one. However, there is a danger here of 'sociologization', that is, of understating the importance of other aspects of the problem, for instance, the psychiatric, axiological, ethical and sociopsychological aspects. The extent to which mental health policy has been embraced can indicate general criteria for health (e.g. life expectancy and population growth), mental health (e.g. level of suicide and level of drug abuse), as well as the actual and perceived levels of criminality. Optimization of all of these indices or, generally speaking, reduction of social tension in different social systems, is attained in different ways.

While in traditional and theocratic societies the place of each person is seen as legitimate, given by God, in democratic societies parliament, press

128

and other social institutions are engaged in more than mere decision making – they act as safety valves for dissent, 'to let off steam':

> The parliamentary institutions, even if they bring harm to legislation and administration of the state ... still have great importance as means of letting out mass and group emotions ... Without such discharging they would have been converted into emotional dynamite [i.e.] resentment. The Russian literature is overfilled with resentment like no other literature of any country. It is a consequence of many ages of oppression of people by tsarist autocracy and of the impossibility to let out emotions because of the absence of parliament and freedom of the press.
>
> (Scheler, 1999: 49)

In authoritarian societies, trust and respect for state institutions are replaced by fear of the prevailing tyranny of force, and the domesticated and subservient parliament and press become immersed in the discourse and folklore of the regime. The level of social tension in such a society is very high, making it aggressive and contributing to militarization. Sport, mass culture and alcohol remain the only outlets.

Aligning the development of legislation and economic reforms with social needs, ensuring a proper standard of living, and developing policy in the fields of education and culture are of fundamental importance. In the case of Russia, which had experienced several revolutionary perestroikas, state concern for the mental health of the population took the form of post-factum formalized reporting rather than any planned and effective concentration of efforts.

Historical epochs and stages of development

It makes sense to discuss a streamlined policy in the field of mental health on the basis of those legislative acts and articles that directly touch upon this field, or otherwise that considerably affect it, as well as of those governmental and departmental acts, that had actually been implemented. In Russia's case it is often said that the salvation from bad laws is their bad implementation. But the latter, regretfully, also affects good laws.

The problem of mental health policy in Russia can be adequately understood only if it is considered in its broad historical context. To this end the following periods of psychiatric service can be identified:

- Pre-Soviet psychiatry
  - Pagan psychiatry
  - Monastic psychiatry (996–1775)
  - Secularization of psychiatry (1715–1775)
  - Institutionalization of psychiatry (1776–1864)

- *Zemstvo* psychiatry (1864–1917)
- Emergence of independent democratic psychiatry (1888–1917)
- Soviet psychiatry
  - Consolidation of professionals (1917–1921)
    The epoch of revolutionary terror and civil war
  - Psychohygienic school and priority of out-patient care (1923–1936)
    The epoch of dispossession of the kulaks (1928–1935)
  - Psychomorphological school and priority of in-patient care (1936–1952)
    The epoch of the Great Terror, wars and repressions
  - Socialist model of psychiatry (1953–1987)
    The epoch of political abuse of psychiatry (1968–1987)
- Post-Soviet psychiatry
  - The epoch of democratic reforms (1988–1994)
  - The epoch of stagnation (from 1995)

The first psychiatric institutions in Russia appeared in 1771–1779 and were under the authority of the Ministry of Police. In Moscow the Pinel reforms were introduced in 1832 by VF Sabler. During that period hospital structure was acknowledged to be the principal prerequisite of medical treatment (Kannabikh, 1929; Yudin, 1951). From 1888 onwards, with the commencement of lectures by SS Korsakov in Moscow, studies in psychiatry became independent from neuropathology.

While the institutionalization of Russian psychiatry as an independent profession had been realized under pressure, heavily shaped by forensic psychiatric concerns under the authority of the Ministry of Police, its institutionalization as a scientific subject was closely connected with the taking off of chains and other measures of non-constraint. The abolition of serfdom in Russia in 1861 served as the social basis for the establishment of scientific psychiatry. Between 1864 and 1870 local self-government [*zemstvos*] was introduced in 31 regions throughout the country, and mental facilities were transferred to these (in St Petersburg and Moscow such transfers took place only in 1887). This marked the most successful epoch of national psychiatry.

For a short time, and despite limited resources and severe shortages of medical personnel, an accessible, first-class – by European standards – health care system was introduced. These developments were achieved by narrowing the range of services and increasing the number of local divisions (from 53 in 1870 up to 2,686 in 1910). By 1880 there were more *zemstvo* doctors in villages than in cities. The convocations of regional medical congresses were formed from 1871 onwards and by the 1880s the All-Russian Pirogov congresses had emerged to take a leading role.

From 1867 onwards psychiatric care was available free of charge to patients in many *zemstvos*. However, the prophylactic orientation of *zemstvo* medicine, with its interference with daily life, did not sit comfortably with the Ministry of Police. Police authorities considered mental institutions as places for isolating violent persons rather than medical establishments, and were in constant conflict with doctors.

In 1891, against a background of counter-reforms (as regards the reform of 1861 and *zemstvo*) a heated debate erupted over the organization of care for the mentally ill in the Moscow *zemstvo* (Yudin, 1951). As part of this debate Yakobiy (1900) proposed a series of principles that became prominent in the 20th century:

- To give preference to treatment and raising the health of the population – rather than guarding it, thus removing psychiatry from administration by the police.
- To institutionalize recently ill patients according to need rather than admitting all patients.
- To organize psychiatric care according to the registration of those needing help rather than on the basis of a general census.
- To use census results to set priorities for hospital locations and sizes (60–200 beds).
- To give preference to decentralization, establishing many small hospitals (for 25 patients) rather than constructing large hospitals.
- To give preference to pavilion-style hospitals rather than those that are barrack-style.
- To provide allowances to the families of the mentally ill who are not admitted to hospital.

In 1911, a draft legislation on the mentally ill (Bazhenov, 1911) was proposed, which, similar to an earlier document in 1887, echoed contemporary psychiatric legislation in other countries. However, the Congress of Psychiatrists withheld approval, despite similar laws having been passed in other countries between 1838 and 1905.

In spite of the epoch of reaction, the last three decades (1888–1917) of the *zemstvo* period saw the flourishing of Russian psychiatry. A fully modern programme of mental health care was established, as was local health care and a scientific community devoted to psychiatry, all independent of government. The extent of these democratic achievements, crowned by the February revolution (February–October 1917), has not been equalled up to the present time.

From the start of World War I the number of hospitals and beds decreased constantly. In 1905 there were 128 mental hospitals (33,607 beds) which amounted to 2.1 beds per 10,000 population; by 1914 this had reduced to 96 hospitals (27,146 beds); and by 1919 the figure was down to 60 hospitals (16,000 beds). By 1922 the number of patients being managed by the mental health system had decreased even more: by 3.2 times in Russia and by 5.7 times in the Ukraine. These figures corresponded to colossal human losses sustained during and following the war years: 2.5 million killed in World War I; 2 million dead of typhoid in 1918–1921, among them victims of the revolutionary terror; 5 million dead of famine in 1921; up to 7 million casualties of the Civil War; and 2 million emigrants. Cities became deserted and in many places the social structure changed, and almost all of the cultural elite was lost. Consequently, the level of mental health care available in 1905 was only again reached in 1935: 102 hospitals (33,772 beds) amounting to 3.1 beds per 10,000 population.

In the early part of the Soviet epoch, up to the revolutionary terror, the field of health policy and mental health actively and forcefully carried out planned measures in accordance with Marxist–Leninist theory, opposing the natural tendencies of development. This grandiose and cruel social experiment sought to enrol the population of a large country in liquidating both the instincts of private property and freedom, and the institutions of family and religion, thus creating a 'new man'. In effect, this movement took on a quasi-religious character. Reporting on family members to the authorities, and raising children from an early age to be part of a collective rather than part of a family, were cultivated. The child labour colonies associated with A Makarenko (1920–1935) became models for other totalitarian regimes.

In 1918 Soviet Russia established the first Ministry of Health in the world. This consisted of both a neuropsychiatric section and a child psychopathology unit. The orientation of prophylactic health care was emphasized, giving priority to the struggle against social diseases (e.g. tuberculosis, venereal diseases, alcoholism). Providing medical care free of charge also became a priority. These considerations were included in the programme of the ruling Russian Communist Party (*Bolsheviki*) in 1919. The article on psychiatric evaluation in the 1919 programme interpreted criteria for 'irresponsibility' in very broad terms, allowing psychiatrists to save many people from execution during the years of the revolutionary terror. At the same time, however, the authorities, including Lenin, used the 'sanitarium' to dispose of political opponents.

In 1921 the central police reception, which since its creation in 1899 had been converted by AN Bernshtein into an exemplary humanistic establishment, was abolished. It was replaced by the Serbski Institute of Forensic Psychiatry, named after an opponent of police psychiatry, but operating under police authority as never before. The first Soviet Institute of Psychiatry, founded in Moscow in 1921, was closed in 1923 after it had rejected the state course for 'specifically Soviet' psychology and psychiatry. PB Gannushkin, who had been head of the central hospital of the country following the demise of Serbski (since 1917), said in 1925 that even his clinic patients were not admitted; they were imprisoned. Between 1924 and 1935, following similar developments in other countries and largely due to the efforts of LM Rozenstein, the psychohygienic trend took hold in Russian psychiatry. Rozenstein established the first state psychoneurological dispensary, providing an out-patient service for the mentally ill, including medical treatment and social help at home. This became the model for analogous facilities all over the country so that by 1929 there were 16 psychoneurological dispensaries. This had grown to 23 by 1931, to 54 by 1940 and to 225 by 1966. Psychoneurological consulting rooms were also being opened in polyclinics. In 1939 there were 458 such consulting rooms and the central dispensary was converted into the Moscow Institute of Psychiatry.

Working on the principle of prophylaxis, researchers began to identify initial forms of mental diseases, and 'mild' and even compensatory conditions, thus widening the borders between schizophrenia and other mental disorders. Randomized evaluations revealed 'neuropsychic diseases' among 54% of workers at some plants and 'neuropsychic indices' among 76% of teachers, shop assistants and so on. Various profiles of neuropsychic disorders were seen as characteristic for different professional groups, with corresponding unhealthy conditions of work, thereby indicating a need for prophylactic measures. Psychohygienic consulting rooms were organized in the plants of big industrial centres, for both intellectual and industrial labour (Yudin, 1951).

Adherents of the psychohygienic school undertook professional selection using psychotechnical methods. As a result of a broad-minded outlook, narcological dispensaries were converted into a section of the Society for Struggle Against Alcoholism, and child preventative out-patient units (dispensaries) were merged with pedological and pedagogical establishments. Complete pedological examination of students was now introduced into secondary schools. However, the theoretical basis of the psychohygienic approach, comprising reflexology, psychoanalysis, pedology and psychotechnics, was destroyed in 1927–1936. Pedology was accused of class bias towards slow students of the proletariat. In 1936 the Moscow and Kharkov Institutes of Psychohygiene were broken up. At the Congress of Psychiatrists in 1936 it was proposed that psychopaths be rehabilitated at the Belomorcanal and that widening the borders of schizophrenia should be considered as 'actually harmful'. Thus, the attempt of the psychohygienic school to take psychoneurological competence out of a narrow circle of defective abnormal patients and to bring it to the mass of the healthy population, and to apply it to the organization of behaviour of a separate personality and to the organization of a concrete environment, conditions of production, labour and way of life, proved to be dangerous for psychiatrists themselves.

Detailed psychopathological descriptions of the files of the Central Dispensary designated for comparison with catamnesis research have been lost. The files were destroyed by the special services because of the danger of Moscow falling to the Germans. Dispensaries were ordered to work in close contact with mental hospitals and to carry on out-patient treatment. As a result, an intermediary form – the half-dispensary or daily out-patient centre for the mentally ill – emerged. Such facilities, the so-called labour prophylactories, were organized in mental hospitals and dispensaries. Some dispensaries began to provide patients with work at home; others, trying to teach independence, gave payment for piece-work.

Established in 1936, the All-Union Society of Neuropathologists and Psychiatrists recommended the following grading system for mental facilities:

- Dispensaries.
- Local hospitals with 100 beds for primary patients.
- Hospitals for long-stay patients.
- Agricultural labour colonies for chronic patients capable of working.
- Houses for invalids of the Narcomsobes (People's Commissariat of Social Welfare) system.

In 1936, various kinds of shock treatment were introduced. Between 1936 and 1952 priority was given to the development of in-patient care, due to the achievements of the psychomorphological (neurological) school in psychiatry.

The politicization of Soviet psychiatry is clearly demonstrated by dramatic changes (in unison with changes of internal political direction) in the evaluation, as irresponsible, persons or psychopaths (from 46.5% in 1922, to 3–4% in 1935–1940), as well as of patients with chronic central nervous system conditions (a two-fold decrease from 1922–1935 to 1936–1945) and of schizophrenic patients (100% until 1933).[1]

These events took place against a background of tremendous human losses. In 1936, in response to the need to raise the birth rate, the family was reinstituted and abortions were banned (they had been allowed in 1917 and became available again from 1955). The mass destruction of the peasantry was undertaken during the period of the psychohygienic movement in psychiatry, with more than seven million perishing due to the artificially created famine, with the dispossession of the kulaks during 1928–1935. This was followed by the epoch of the Great Terror. By the end of the 1930s the number of inmates in concentration camps had reached 10 million. A further 27 million perished in World War II. Mass repressions also continued after the War. During these years the combined effect of the defeat of proponents of genetics, the ascendancy of Pavlov's ideas and the

---

[1] A clear indication of why the borders of schizophrenia were narrowed.

contentious Doctors' Plot in 1952 when some doctors, most of whom were Jewish, were accused of poisoning, (Clarfield, 2002) led to the lowering of medical standards, primitivization of manuals on psychiatry, the destruction of many volumes of important works such as *The Experience of the Great Patriotic War* and undermining of the neurological (psychomorphological) direction in psychiatry.

While the epoch of what will be referred to as the 'socialist model of psychiatry' (1953–1988) is usually described as an apologetic one, this was in fact effective for the system, providing a range of medical services free of charge, supporting the right of the mentally ill to additional dwelling space (for instance, a private room) and influencing labour legislation, regulating hiring and dismissal from offices for the benefit of workers, and so on. In 1953 the Statute on Psychoneurological Dispensaries in regions, cities and districts was issued. This inherited much from the experience of the psychohygienic school, including: an emphasis on the early detection of the mentally ill; provision of district level dispensary care; organization of subsidiary farms and medical-industrial workshops; assistance with occupational training and obtaining work; provision of child and adolescent consulting rooms, as well as psychotherapeutic and logopaedic consulting rooms; and population-based education on basic hygiene and sanitary norms. In the years 1972–1979 psychoneurological dispensaries or dispensary units were opened in cities where the population was greater than 200,000. Under this system a district psychiatrist was designated for every 40,000 adult population and every 30,000 children. However, during the 1980s this changed to one psychiatrist for every 30,000 adults and every 20,000 children. As a result, the number of district psychiatrists in Russia increased from 4,633 in 1985 to 5,775 in 1989 (Kazakovtsev, 1996).

The negative experience of the Soviet repressive model of treatment of alcoholism in the period 1967–1990 is instructive. Medico-vocational prophylactic establishments (LTP) existed in the system of the Interior Ministry. These were actually labour camps where involuntary treatment was administered. Since 1975, narcological care has been separated as an independent service with a network of narcological dispensaries. However, along with sobering-up stations and LTP these soon acquired a negative reputation. The narcological dispensaries were not observing confidentiality, thefts were occurring in the sobering-up stations and LTP services were fulfilling the function of 'purification' of the population. Against this background the grotesque anti-alcohol campaign of 1985–1987 did not prevent an increase in the number of alcoholics, although there was an almost four-fold reduction in alcoholic psychoses in the same period. The tendency for alcoholism to spread and intensify has continued, and since 1985 there has been a substantial increase in narcomania. A high rate of suicide, especially among those in the internal security forces, gave impetus to the creation of a suicide service.

Such was the contradictory nature of Soviet ideology that declarations on 'the most humane health care system in the world' sat alongside secret lists of ecological and professional harmfulness, numerous catastrophes such as Chernobyl, the banning of open dosimeters, and so on.

The history of Russian psychiatry and all its achievements took place under the extremely difficult conditions of a police regime. The years of Soviet power were characterized by unprecedented cruelty and mass character assassination, denouncing, control over ideological purity, and constant interference by the Party into science, art and private life. Under these conditions, mental institutions proved to be sanctuaries, where one could survive. The overthrow of Stalin's cult had engendered a free-thinking generation of men and women 'of the sixties', who embraced the human rights movement. On the initiative of the (then) KGB chief, Yuri Andropov, from the early 1960s, but especially from 1969, mental hospitals were used to discredit and suppress this movement. The fulfilment of such a police order was made easier by the preventative attitude of Soviet psychiatry and the sophisticated clinicism of the Snezhevski school with its hyperdiagnostics of schizophrenia. As was the case in the time of Arakcheev (1815–1825), patients were being admitted to mental hospitals with a note in the case history 'discharge by the order' rather than the formerly accepted note 'after recovery'.

It was not surprising that psychiatric registration frightened people, for registration in a psychoneurological dispensary, even for primary patients, was connected with the serious curtailment of civil rights (including travel abroad, issue of driving licences, applying for a job, and entering higher educational establishments). Being removed from the register was immeasurably more difficult than being placed on it. Irrespective of health condition the patient had to visit a psychiatrist twice annually, otherwise an employee of the dispensary would be sent to the patient's home. A large part of the population was required to produce a certificate of 'non-registration' in relation to mental health. The widespread use of criminal prosecution for the 'distribution of information discrediting the Soviet state system' led to the prosecution of a large number of persons with mental disorders. Inspection of the special mental hospitals revealed that at least one in nine of these in St Petersburg admitted at different times over 2,000 people for political reasons. Moreover, data on the Kazan mental hospital, the largest of these institutions and specially intended for political patients, has been concealed up until now. Information on these mass repressive practices undoubtedly contributed to the spread of the anti-psychiatry movement around the world. This international resonance made the observation of human rights one of the priority conditions for the

Soviet Union's favoured-nation treatment and for its integration into the world economic community. In what was a characteristic 'revolution from above', the transition to a new epoch in psychiatry was initiated in the time of Soviet power.

The recent situation

The year 1988 was marked by two important events. The Statute on conditions and order of rendering psychiatric care was adopted, which included for the first time a formulation of patients' rights. In addition, regulations governing the observation, care and control of patients were also developed. In an initiative marking the beginnings of a programme of humanization, special mental hospitals for patients with criminal records were transferred from the Interior Ministry to the Ministry of Health. Nevertheless, these were belated half-measures, dissatisfaction with which led in 1989 to the founding of the Independent Psychiatric Association (IPA) of Russia. The priorities of this non-governmental, professional and human rights organization were based on an analysis of the unprecedented scale of abuses associated with psychiatry in Russia. Accordingly, the IPA adopted the following priorities: return to the phenomenological method under the editorship of Jaspers, adoption of the Law on Psychiatric Care, and partial removal of psychiatry from state control.

The further development of Russian psychiatry is directly connected with movement in this direction. In 1989 criminal articles on 'anti-Soviet agitation and propaganda' (Art. 70 of the Criminal Code) and 'distribution of deliberately false fabrications, discrediting the Soviet state and social system' (Art. 190-1 of the Criminal Code) were abrogated and people convicted under those articles were freed. In what amounted to an indirect acknowledgement of the large-scale abuse of psychiatry, changing the interpretation of social danger and softening discrimination against the mentally ill led to about two million people being removed from dispensary registration in 1989–1990. In 1990 the first version of the Law on Psychiatric Care was developed. The attempted anti-reform uprising led to the revolution of 1991.

The collapse of the Soviet empire was followed by total crisis. This involved the destruction of political institutions, curtailing of production, migration of the population, loss of savings of the population, non-payment of wages, decline of living standards, enormous contrasts between poverty and wealth and, as a result, a powerful leap of social tension and resentment in society, xenophobia and extremism. The collapse of Soviet ideology, widespread uncertainty, corruption in all echelons and branches of power, undisclosed political killings, and an outdated judicial system have provoked distrust and disrespect for the existing legal and social order, and a lack of perspective resulting in anomy and the need for religion. Psychiatric services became disorganized due to the destruction of the former system of social-labour rehabilitation, lack of funds, outflow of the best personnel, and the catastrophic worsening of the indices of physical and mental health. Life expectancy dropped sharply and decline in birthrate crossed the critical line. The number of successful suicides in 1991–1995 increased by 1.6 times, having reached 41.4 per 100,000 of population (when 20 per 100,000 is considered critical). In a number of places the suicide rate is extremely high, for instance, in Ural, Povolzhye and Siberia the rate is 65–81 suicides per 100,000, and in the republic of Komi and Udmurtia 150–180 per 100,000. In the years 1991–1997, the incidence of alcoholism increased by 25% and alcoholic psychoses increased six-fold in adults and nine-fold in adolescents; the incidence of narcomania, mainly among young persons, increased seven-fold and the number of socially dangerous acts committed by the mentally ill more than doubled (Gurovitch, 2001; Kazakovtsev, 1998; Krasnov, 2001; Yastrebov, 1999).

The epoch of democratic reforms in the field of psychiatry has been marked by a number of big landmarks. These are:

- Adoption of the Law on Psychiatric Care (1 January 1993).
- Return to international standards for diagnosing schizophrenia, and transition to ICD-10.
- De-monopolization and de-centralization of psychiatry, in particular, priority given to financing regional programmes and transfer to financing concrete medical services, but not traditional upkeep of establishments.
- Reforming the Ministry of Health and its psychiatric department, and getting rid of the most extreme figures of the former leadership (1990–1991).
- Creation of the *Independent Psychiatric Journal* (since December, 1991), through which the professional community acquired the voice of freedom, was able to state its programme of action and to clearly demarcate the productive and destructive tendencies of the anti-psychiatric movement.
- Appearance of a great number of new psychiatric journals instead of a single one, as in the Soviet epoch.
- Foundation of a substantial number of non-professional non-governmental organizations, working in the sphere of mental health.
- Inclusion into the new Criminal Code of 1996 the norms of diminished responsibility and involuntary out-patient observation and treatment.

The first Russian Law on Psychiatric Care and Guarantees of Citizens'

Rights in its Provision formulated inadmissibility of any restriction of rights on the sole basis of psychiatric diagnosis, dispensary observation or admission to a mental hospital. Visiting a psychiatrist has become a confidential matter between the health professional and the patient. The basic principles are the principle of voluntary visits to a psychiatrist and clear-cut regulation of grounds for involuntary hospitalization, which is now sanctioned by the courts. The Law has introduced public control over the observation of patients' rights. In spite of the fact that some articles of the Law have remained as declarations only, the adoption of the Law is an important accomplishment, giving impetus to the development of the rudiments of medical law in Russia. Again the route was taken to the social-medical (but not purely medical) model of psychiatric care, promoting it to the population and giving priority to out-patient care in which paternalism is replaced with a partnership (Kabanov, 1998). The name 'dispensary', which had been compromised, was changed to 'mental health centre' in many regions (although not in Moscow). In general, polyclinics or psychoneurological consulting rooms were opened, various forms of half-day out-patient units were created, various methods of sociotherapy were established and psychotherapeutic services began to develop. Psychologists were given the right to work in the psycho-correctional area. Faculties of clinical psychology were opened not only in humanitarian universities, but also in medical institutions. The profession of social worker was introduced and the corresponding faculties were opened. Paid services were introduced and the strict territorial principle for rendering medical care was eased. Various forms of co-operation with religious organizations developed and various non-governmental organizations, self-help organizations and associations of relatives of the mentally ill began to emerge.

The epoch of the stagnation of democratic reforms dates from the start of the war in Chechnya in 1995. Secrecy increased and statements denying the abuses of psychiatry in the past became more frequent. Once again psychiatry was used for non-medical purposes: this time for the suppression of various religious organizations. As a pretext it was asserted that 'totalitarian sects' inflict serious damage to the mental health of believers. In spite of the fact that such data had been disavowed by both victims and all-Russian psychiatric societies as scientifically unfounded, the Ministry of Health together with the Interior Ministry continued to disseminate this information throughout the country. The offices of the Public Prosecutor from St Petersburg to Magadan were involved in bringing numerous actions against religious organizations, infringing the rights of believers by the imposition of 'care'.

The low priority given to mental health in Russia is vividly demonstrated in the following situations:

- In the early 1990s in some regions the heavy paternalism of psychiatric institutions was replaced by connivance, and the interests of the mentally ill ceased to be protected, contributing to mass abuses of the privatization of apartments and resulting in many mentally ill people joining the army of the homeless.
- The chief psychiatrist of the Ministry of Health of the Russian Federation (RF) in 1996 admitted that Russia lagged behind the countries which took part in the psychiatric reform, by at least half a century. Mental hospitals are very often located in former barracks, concentration camps, prisons and monasteries.
- The federal programme 'Urgent measures for improving psychiatric care', adopted by the RF Government for 1995–1996, was financed by only 0.2% of the gross national product, and was not realized.
- In 1997–1998, as a result of a gross lack of funds in many mental hospitals, patients were starving. For instance, in the Moscow region, mental hospitals were receiving 7–8% of the sum needed for medicines and 20–25% of the funds required for food. Both psychiatric societies and the Chamber for Human Rights expressed alarm, but the authorities failed to address the issue adequately.
- The Law on Narcotic Drugs and Psychotropic Substances, in force since January 1998, which had been worked out by the Interior Ministry in spite of protests by the psychiatric organizations, was purely oriented to using force and police methods for solving the problems of substance abuse. This law erased the border between toxicomania and narcomania, put up obstacles to obtaining psychotropic medicines, and banned treatment of narcomania outside state institutions, which are financed by 4% of required funding, thus contributing to the situation where 70% of those convicted for 'drug trafficking' are common users.
- Although religious 'sects' provide the most effective help in respect of the national disaster of narcomania, since 1995 authorities have been trying to close them under the pretext of 'inflicting damage to mental health'. This is a consequence of the interlocking of the state and the Russian Orthodox Church.
- Between 1989 and 1995 the number of convicts increased constantly, reaching 720–780 per 100,000 population in 1998, a figure that is 7–13 times higher than in European countries. However, only 12–16% of convicts are actually dangerous. Since 1992, the use of torture and the training of special forces to deal with convicts have become commonplace. Neither the new Criminal Code of 1997, nor the transfer of penitentiary establishments from the system of the Interior Ministry to the Ministry of Justice in 1998 changed the situation substantially. In Russian legislation there is no definition of 'torture'. There is an absence of state criminal law policy; the Soviet punitive tradition is

largely being maintained, and moves to partially decentralize the administration of penitentiary institutions and to introduce judicial and public control are being opposed (Abramkin, 1999).

The current situation (21st century)

Russia's population is currently 146.3 million, of whom 44 million live below the poverty line and the official subsistence minimum. The country is ranked 47th among developing countries on the 'well-being' index, i.e. the degree of balance achieved between development indices in economic, social and information spheres (China is ranked 46th and India 49th). Gross domestic product (GDP) amounts to 10 trillion rubles. In 2001 health care in Russia was allocated 2% (200 billion rubles) of GDP, of which psychiatry received 0.13% (13 billion rubles) or 6.5% of the overall health care allocation (Kazakovtsev, 1996; 1998). While expert evaluations indicate that 14% of the population needs psychiatric care (Rotshtein et al., 2001), only 2.6% receive it. There are 173,400 beds in psychiatric institutions. For the first time since 1995 the number of registered patients with non-psychotic disorders outnumbered the number of patients with psychoses and feeble-mindedness (1.6:1). Moreover, 10% of the population needs narcological care but only 1.6% receives it (270,000 drug addicts and 2,111,000 chronic alcoholics). While the rate of increase of narcomania has abated in recent years, this nevertheless continues to increase by 12.5% per annum (Koshkina, 2001). The number of psychiatrists is currently over 15,000; there are more than 2,000 psychotherapists and 4,000 narcologists.

The 'strengthening of vertical administration' by the new authorities has contributed to the restoration of an authoritarian style within and beyond the law enforcement departments. The Serbski State Centre of Social and Forensic Psychiatry is now a more influential force in psychiatry than at any time in the past. The independent mass media, the Chamber for Human Rights and the Pardon Commission of the President have been dissolved. Political and non-governmental structures are being enlarged and organized in ways that are pro-state. The corruption and criminalization of power structures have reached an unprecedented scale. Gross violation of human rights in Chechnya by the law enforcement departments has had a profound demoralizing influence. All participants in the war in Chechnya (over one million servicemen in the federal forces alone) need psychological rehabilitation (Linnikova, 1998). The number of refugees and involuntary migrants stands at about 8.6 million and only 760,000 of these have managed to gain refugee status. In 2000 the number of heinous and extremely grave crimes increased 1.5 times in 17 regions (Lukashevski,

2000). However, while the substantial strengthening of authoritarian tendencies has slowed the process of reforms, this has not stopped altogether.

Meanwhile, the main psychiatric reforms are taking place in the regions, rather than in the capital cities. These regional reforms are characterized by their gratifying variety, independence and innovation, rather than the mechanical copying of foreign experience, which is usually ineffective. In some regions a team method of care has been introduced, constructive cooperation with various religious organizations has been secured, and professional organizations, trying to influence the situation in psychiatry, are being established.

The number and variety of commercial non-governmental structures rendering medical care is increasing; new forms of education, in particular, in juridical universities and establishments of the Interior Ministry system are being introduced. Another gratifying factor is the substantially increased role of the individual. The legal appointment of representatives of non-governmental organizations in certification, licensing and other commissions is a substantial achievement, although it has not yet been possible to realize these rights. It is important that even under present conditions society is able to exert some form of influence over mental health policy. The very existence and successful activities of the IPA of Russia testifies to the end of the total state control of psychiatry. The IPA of Russia, along with human rights organizations and journalists, exercise civil control over the observation of the Universal Declaration on Human Rights and other international pacts ratified by Russia, including the package of federal laws concerning psychiatric care and the Madrid Ethical Code (Savenko, 1999). The commissions of the IPA of Russia periodically visit all mental hospitals for patients with criminal records. The first Congress of Child Psychiatrists, held in 2001, which demanded restoration of the profession of child psychiatry (dissolved in 1995) and various legal acts on child facilities, have highlighted this important area of mental health care. Juvenile justice is developing. The alternative drafts of a law on psychotherapeutical care have also been worked out.

Nevertheless, in spite of the catastrophic situation, psychiatric care and mental health have not been taken up as priority themes in post-Soviet Russia. The policy of a state reveals itself not in declarations, but in actual levels of funding provided to services. Unfortunately, the funding provided to the Russian mental health system is much less than required. There should be differentiation between the level of need, the extent of planning, the services provided, and what actually reaches the patient. Nevertheless, the funding situation for the up-keep and treatment of the mentally ill has stabilized compared to the situation faced in 1994–1998. Very significantly, the new Ministry of Health strategy for reorganization of the network of psychiatric institutions provides for earmarked funding for each region. However, this programme was scheduled to commence not earlier than 2002.

The priority tasks for the organization of mental health care include: inclusion in mainstream health services, decentralization of administration, economic independence, the working out of standards of quality of care, the staged transfer to a system of health insurance, the development of self-help groups and so on. However, current mental health policy lacks a sophisticated appreciation of the complexities to be managed at the government level. Even in the face of the catastrophic demographic and ecological situations confronting Russia, the health of the population has not been made a policy priority. The eternal value of the family is not being cultivated and some non-governmental organizations working in this area (e.g. family, Church of Unification, and so on) are being prosecuted for ideological reasons. The publicizing of legal data on ecological crimes committed by the Ministry of Defence has led to the prosecution of a number of scientists and military journalists. Moreover, the catastrophic situation with social diseases – tuberculosis, alcoholism, narcomania, syphilis and HIV/AIDS – is closely connected with the police tradition of repression (e.g. the incidence of tuberculosis in pre-trial detention centres is 58 times greater than outside prison; the law on narcotic drugs and psychotropic substances has been framed as a 'war on users', but not on drug traffickers). Propaganda on a healthy lifestyle in the mass media has been limited to efforts to shift youth preferences from strong beverages to beer.

While the sociology of medicine has begun to develop, the sociology of psychiatry and social psychiatry is becoming the monopoly of the heavily politicized Serbski State Centre of Social and Forensic Psychiatry. As a result, understanding of the recent situation and the programme of planned responses lacks the systematic interdisciplinary character, scale and determination required by the severity of the problems faced. Attempts to improve legal regulation are being undermined by the slowing down of judicial reform, and also by the ideological character and low level of law making (e.g. discrepancy between, and absence of, guarantees that laws will be observed), absence of independent judicial power, and corresponding to all of these, lack of a sense of justice (e.g. lack of belief in, and respect for, laws). However, the end result of all efforts is determined by the everyday consciousness and the 'real-life world' of ordinary individuals and small groups, i.e. things that go without saying in real-life practice. For instance, rather than the 'spiritual' efforts of Alcoholics Anonymous, the suggestive-stress method of 'coding' is seen as the most effective treatment method for alcoholism, and the country's leading intellectuals prefer healers to scientific medicine, at least with respect to psychiatry. This testifies to the decline of professional prestige.

Examination of mental health policy in the context of the problem of social control is often limited by adherence to a regulative-adaptive framework which assumes a model of a *stabilizing* system of self-regulation of the homoeostasis type. This gross simplification is especially evident in periods of crisis when the influence of minor factors is amplified and the role of the individual as a passive object of control is highlighted. The new general scientific paradigm advocates the use of a model of a *monitoring* system of self-regulation of the homeorhesis type, allowing consideration of the direction and content of necessary changes. This shift from a stabilizing model to a monitoring one requires the system to be refined. What is needed is a qualitative leap in its maturation from protective to defensive mechanisms – in the organism (Goldstein, 1940), and from authoritarian to democratic – in society (Lewin et al., 1939). The widely accepted sociological tenet that the reinforcement of police repressive measures leads to the strengthening, not weakening, of social deviance is generally ignored in Russia. Much-needed tolerance, consensus and compromise are replaced by parodies, and appropriated into devices of the political game. Once again the abuses of the past are denied (Dmitrieva, 2001).

It is apparent that the major disputes surrounding mental health policy stem from the different priorities given to personality, society and state. The new democratic order of priorities, written into the Constitution, remains an empty declaration. The life and health of the individual are, as before, nothing in comparison to the interests of the empire. The prevailing concepts of 'society', 'state' and 'politics' differ from those in Western-style liberal democracies to such a degree that they are rather homonymous and lead to confusion. In Russia the struggle for state law continues to fall well short of the legal state, the more so to a democratic one. Formation of civil society is at an embryonic stage. However, it should be noted that a similar situation in the years 1888–1917 did not hamper the most successful period of development of Russian psychiatry.

In spite of the evident failure of a state model of securing mental health, this approach continues to dominate the theory and practice of Russian psychiatry, health care and political leadership as a whole. Although the great potential for the self-organization of society is starting to be recognized, this continues to be overshadowed by the tradition of deeply felt distrust for and suspicion of unplanned and uncontrollable processes. As a result, non-governmental initiatives are again replaced by imitations imposed from above and thus have little impact. Indeed, the problem of mental health is of little interest to the state authorities, except for those who are mental health specialists. Initiatives, when they occur, are largely limited to public relations activities. Moreover, the mental health theme is often exploited demagogically to legally justify the introduction of censorship and other repressive measures (e.g. Draft Law on Informational

Psychological Security and Appeal to the RF President of the representative of Russia in the World Health Organization)[2].

History indicates that Soviet psychiatry, which had proclaimed prophylaxis as its principal credo and the main direction of its efforts, and which was well positioned to capitalize on the unique possibilities before it, demonstrated between the periods 1923–1935 and 1969–1988 the serious shortcomings of that direction. In 1935–1936 the psychiatrization of social life produced sharp dissatisfaction with the authorities because of the interference in production. In 1988–1989 widespread discontent led to a general protest supported by democratic countries against the violation of human rights. The double-edged and ambivalent character of the prophylactic orientation, as this unfolded at various times in the history of Russian psychiatry, presents lessons that are broadly instructive. In Russia it led to a situation in which mental health policy has been limited by the organization of psychiatric services. Since 1995 certain aspects of the prophylactic orientation have again taken on a negative character, being heavily determined by the political background. There is a danger that seeking to expand the scope of professional competence in pursuit of financing will lead to overestimation of the numbers requiring psychiatric care, widening of the definition of post-traumatic stress, expanding the notions of 'self-destructive' and 'dependent' behaviour, and erasing the borders of serious disorders requiring first aid. Finally, the psychiatrization of social life inevitably draws psychiatry into the realm of politics, resulting in constant attempts to use it for non-medical purposes.

Civil society is rapidly developing in all directions in Russia. The problem of psychiatric care, indeed also of mental health, is that it is vividly evident that progressive reform is not possible without the mobilization of the forces of society.

Experience

The priority of the state over the individual in the mentality of the leaders of state psychiatry was clearly revealed in the dispute of 2000–2001 in the Ministry of Health Commission on changes and amendments to the Law on Psychiatric Care. The majority of Commission members – leading psychiatrists of the state centres of psychiatry – had been trying to reserve the Ministry's right to adopt legal (not only departmental) acts and to sharply broaden the grounds for involuntary hospitalization, removing the restrictive definition in the term 'direct danger'. This was rejected due to the opinion of the IPA of Russia (IPA, 1999), supported

[2] The Appeal was made public at the meeting of the Scientific Council of the Institute for Study and Prophylactics of Terrorism in 2001.

by juridical experts. The preferred wording of the IPA was included in the final version of the draft law (24 September 2001).

The ideological nature of struggles surrounding mental health was vividly demonstrated at a trial in Chelyabinsk in 2000, one of many which have taken place since 1995. The General Prosecutor's Office tried in legal form to impose a ban on the Society of Enlightenment (KARP), founded by the Church of Unification on the grounds of the 'harmful effect on the subconscious level of anti-narcomania lectures'. Due to the intervention of the IPA the legal action of the General Prosecutor's Office was turned down (Savenko, 2001).

To date a state service for protection of patients' rights, envisaged in the Law of 1993, has not been established and an attempt by the IPA of Russia to create such a service in the non-governmental sector in 2001 was refused by the Moscow Health Committee, which labelled the initiative 'untimely'. The IPA continues to pursue this initiative in the Moscow region, which, unlike Moscow, represents the situation in the country.

As in the past, the situation in Russia is characterized by the Interior Ministry's use of various forms of torture, in particular, detention for six months or longer in pre-trial detention centres and temporary isolation wards. Even following humanization of the penitentiary legislation in March 2001 these establishments remain overcrowded by two to three times. Cells intended for 10 persons often hold up to 30 and this has previously been as high as 50. Inmates are forced to sleep in shifts. The poor quality of the air is such that inmates perish due to lack of oxygen, and tuberculosis can develop after only a few months. The pre-trial detention centres in Moscow are the most overcrowded in Russia, being intended for 7,000 places they are filled with 17–21,000 prisoners. In 2001 some 170 detention centres throughout the country held 220,000 detainees in facilities intended for only 112,000. In 1998, 320,000 detainees had been in custody and the building programme for pre-trial detention centres for 1992–1996 received only 1–3% of the originally planned amount. Such are the conditions of detention of those who have not yet been sentenced in court (Abramkin, 1999).

Summary

Mental health policy in Russia has always been limited by the organization of psychiatric care. Its division into periods and its description over the last century reveals some large-scale homological cycles of prophylactic orientation, i.e. attempts to bring a prophylactic focus into mental health policy. Due to the authoritarian nature of successive political regimes in the country, all such attempts have led to negative outcomes. In the contemporary situation mental health policy is again being defined by the priorities of the state, with little opportunity for society or the individual to exert influence. And judging from the funding allocation, the fundamental importance of this area of public policy is not being recognized in spite of the catastrophic indices of mental health and the disastrous narcological, ecological and demographic situations currently facing Russia. Meanwhile, without the involvement of society it is unlikely that the state will be able to solve these problems. While the process of reforms has slowed, it nevertheless continues, with the most positive outcomes being evident in various regions. It is clear that giving health and mental health priority in state policy would provide a strong foundation for solving many other problems in a timely and constructive way.

References

Abramkin VF (Ed.) (1999) Person (a Man) and Prison. Moscow: Centre for Criminal Reform.

Bazhenov NN (1911) Draft Legislation on the Mentally Ill and Explanatory Note to it. Moscow: City Printing House.

Clarfield AM (2002) The Soviet 'Doctors' Plot' – 50 years on. British Medical Journal, 325: 1487–1489.

Dmitrieva TB (2001) Alliance of Law and Mercy. Moscow: Science.

Goldstein K (1940) On two forms of adjustment to defects. Neuropathology and Psychiatry, 6: 116–24.

Gurovitch IY (2001) Mental health of population and psychiatric care in Russia. Social and Clinical Psychiatry, 1: 9–15.

IPA (1999) The IPA's own opinion on the draft of changes and amendments to the Federal Law 'On Psychiatric Care'. Independent Psychiatric Journal, 1: 82–83; and 2000 1: 44–50.

Kabanov MM (1998) Psycho-social Rehabilitation and Social Psychiatry. St. Petersburg: Medicine.

Kannabikh Y (1929) History of Psychiatry. Moscow: State Medicine Publishing House.

Kazakovtsev BA (1996) Organization of Psychiatric Care. Moscow: RF Mental Health Printing House.

Kazakovtsev BA (1998) Development of psychiatric care in Russia. Independent Psychiatric Journal, 2: 9–12.

Koshkina EA (2001) Extent of narcological diseases in the RF according to official statistical data. Questions of Narcology, 3: 61–7.

Krasnov VN (2001) Protection of mental health is a common responsibility. Social and Clinical Psychiatry, 2: 5–6.

Lewin K, Lippit R, White R (1939) Patterns of aggressive behavior in experimentally created social climates. Journal of Social Psychology, 10: 271–99.

Linnikova II (Ed.) (1998) On Violations of Human Rights in Russia. Moscow: Human Rights.

Lukashevski SM (Ed.) (2000) Human Rights in Regions of the RF. V. 1. Moscow: International Helsinki Federation for Human Rights, ZAO RITS 'ZATSEPA'.

Rotshtein VG, Yastrebov VS, Bogdan MN, Seiku YV (2001) Current system of psychiatric care: Epidemiological aspect. Korsakov Journal of Neuropathology and Psychiatry, 4:42–7.

Savenko YS (1999) Psychiatry and human rights. Independent Psychiatric Journal, 1: 15–20, 14–16, 81–4.

Savenko YS (2001) Expansion of ideology to mental health. Independent Psychiatric Journal, 2: 50–7.

Scheler M (1999) Das Ressentiment im Aufbau der Moralen. St. Petersburg: St. Petersburg University.

Yakobiy PI (1900) Administrative Psychiatry. Orel: Gubernski Administration Printing House.

Yastrebov VS (1999) Organization of psychiatric care. Manual on Psychiatry. Vol. 1. Moscow: Medicine. pp. 329–55.

Yudin TI (1951) Studies of History of National Psychiatry. Moscow: MEDGIZ.

CHAPTER NINE

Mental health policy in China: The persecution of Falun Gong

VIVIANA GALLI AND SUNNY YANG LU

Note. The views expressed in this article do not represent any group or association.

Introduction

The brutal persecution of Falun Gong has been steadily escalating over the last few years. Tens of millions of peaceful Falun Gong practitioners are under severe mental pressure, illegal detention, heavy forced labour, and physical and psychological torture. The political, social and mental control by the Jiang Zemin regime during this massive persecution is unprecedented, and one of the worst human rights violations in Chinese history. Jiang has tried to hide the true nature and scope of the persecution of Falun Gong, not wanting the world to understand that the entire campaign has been built upon lies and fear in order to mobilize and consolidate his own political power. Indeed, many analysts argue that the persecution has little or nothing to do with the nature of Falun Gong itself, but has merely been used by Jiang to solidify his own political power base.

A new round of escalation of the persecution is spreading in China. It has been reported that orders from the top are to 'kill without mercy' Falun Gong practitioners, and that police have been ordered to 'shoot on sight' anyone posting or handing out Falun Gong materials (Falun Dafa Information Center, 2002a).

The International Education Development at the United Nations has stated:

> In our investigation, the only deaths have been at the hands of the Chinese authorities; families have been broken up as family members have been detained, forced to flee, or been killed by the regime; people have been broken down, not by Falun Gong, but by extreme torture, incarceration in mental hospitals with brutal treatment, hard labor in camps and other such practices.
>
> (International Education Development, 2001)

This very dark chapter in Chinese history began July 1999 with the persecution of Falun Gong. The Chinese government has been using all means at its disposal to 'eradicate' this peaceful practice. Over 510 deaths have been verified since the persecution began. However, government officials inside China reported in October 2001 that the actual death toll at that time exceeded 1,600. Hundreds of thousands of innocent Chinese citizens from all socioeconomic levels have been detained, with more than 100,000 sentenced to forced labour camps without trial, and more than 1,000 involuntarily admitted to mental health facilities (Falun Dafa Information Center, 2002b). Children, schoolteachers, judges, physicians, nurses, high-ranking officials, leading scientists, Communist Party members, military personnel, farmers and just ordinary people who used to meet in public parks to practise a traditional self-healing art have been deprived of their most basic human rights. What is their crime?

Falun Gong, also known as Falun Dafa, is an ancient practice for the mind and the body. It consists of meditation and exercises with teachings based on the universal principles of 'Truthfulness-Compassion-Tolerance'. Falun Gong was taught in private for thousands of years before being made public in 1992 by Li Hongzhi. While Falun Gong has roots in traditional Chinese culture, it is distinct and separate from other practices in China, such as the religions of Buddhism and Taoism. Since its introduction in 1992, Falun Gong quickly spread by word of mouth throughout China, and is now practised in over 50 countries (Falun Dafa.org, 2002).

In the spring of 1999 the government estimated that as many as 100 million people in China were practising Falun Gong. China's President Jiang Zemin outlawed the peaceful practice in July 1999. Fearing something that could touch the hearts and minds of a greater number of citizens than are members of the Communist Party, Jiang began the persecution. The subsequent abuse of psychiatry in the persecution of Falun Gong is simply the most extreme and revealing way in which the campaign against Falun Gong has been an attack on what is sane and healthy. Jiang has used propaganda to twist the minds of the Chinese people, making them unable to tell good from bad. He has enforced a comprehensive information blockade to keep any truth from reaching the Chinese people from outside, or the truth of this evil persecution from reaching the world at large. He has employed the extraordinary and comprehensive tools of social control available to the Communist Party to enforce the lessons of his propaganda, and to substitute the 'party line' for any individual voice of conscience. He has used hideous tortures to attempt to force all Falun Gong practitioners to renounce what they know to be true, quietly imprisoning, torturing and even murdering those who practise it. He has abused psychopharmacology and other tools of psychiatry to attempt to 'eradicate' the very mind and will of those practitioners who resist being 'transformed'. In short, in his persecution of Falun Gong, Jiang Zemin has attempted to plunge the entire Chinese nation into a kind of nightmare world, in which all values are reversed, and torment is brought down on those who attempt to assert what is true and healthy.

Historical background

Falun Gong had not always been the object of enmity of the Chinese government. In 1993 at the Oriental Health Expo in Beijing, Falun Gong was recognized as the 'Star Qigong School' and Li Hongzhi received the Award for Advancing Boundary Science and Qigong Master most Acclaimed by the Masses. Li Hongzhi was also awarded the Honour Certificate Conferred by a Foundation under the Ministry of Public Security of China in December 1993. The Ministry of Public Security of China published a report in the newspaper in September 1993 and a thank-you letter was issued from the foundation under the same ministry in August 1993 (Falun Dafa, Clearwisdom, 2002a). Before the persecution many newspapers and magazine articles listed the numerous health benefits of practising Falun Gong and praised Falun Gong for the money its practitioners saved the government due to a reduction in health care needs.

In 1998, there were five large-scale health surveys of 37,645 Falun Gong practitioners in four different areas in China. The results indicated an overall improvement rate of multiple diseases of 98.7% and a cure rate of 72%. Included among other benefits were better mental health and an anti-ageing effect (He Mai, 2002). As late as 1999, a Chinese official told the US News and World Report that the Premier Zhu Rongji was 'very happy' with the money saved by the Chinese government due to the practice of 'Falun Gong and other types of Qigong' (Fang, 1999).

By the end of 1998, the Chinese government's own estimate was that 70–100 million people in China had taken up the practice. After 50 years of being in power there were only 55 million Communist Party members. Falun Gong had become 'the largest voluntary organization in China, larger even than the Communist Party' (Fang, 1999). On 25 April 1999, preceding the official ban of Falun Gong, there was a peaceful gathering of 10,000 Falun Gong practitioners outside the Office for Making Appeals in Beijing. The crowd was so large that it ended up encircling Zhongnanhai, the compound where the Communist Party leadership lives, a few hundred metres away from the Appeal Office. These 10,000 had come to request the release of 45 practitioners who had been arbitrarily detained by the police in Tianjin two days before. Premier Zhu Rongji personally came out to meet with practitioners and the situation was peacefully resolved by that evening. To many people in China who knew of this event, this set a good example of co-operation between responsible citizens and their government to resolve a difficult issue. However, President Jiang Zemin single-handedly issued a ban of Falun Gong. According to sources inside the Chinese government, he said, 'No measures are too excessive' to wipe out Falun Gong (Johnson, 2000a). It is no secret that several Politburo members thought the president had used the wrong tactics. 'By unleashing a Mao-style movement, Jiang is forcing senior cadres to pledge allegiance to his line,' said a Party veteran. 'This will boost Jiang's authority – and may give him enough momentum to enable him to dictate events at the pivotal 16th Communist Party Congress next year' (Wo-Lap Lam, 2001).

On 7 June 1999, about a month before the suppression of Falun Gong began, the President circulated a letter entitled 'Comrade Jiang Zemin's speech at a meeting of the Politburo of the Central Committee regarding handling and resolving the Falun Gong issue without delay'. This letter established the suppression policy to be used against Falun Gong and by 10 June the Chinese Communist Party Central Committee officially set up an office for the 'leadership group' and named it the 'Head Office for Handling the Falun Gong Issue', also called the '610 office'. The 610 office is an agency specifically created to persecute Falun Gong, with absolute power over each level of administration in the Party and all other political and judiciary systems. The rapid increase in deaths over the past year is a direct result of the orders from the 610 office (Falun Dafa Information Center, 2002c).

Contemporary situation

Social control through mind control

The rule of the Communist Party over the past half-century in China is entirely built on the foundation of the tight mind control of the now 1.3 billion Chinese people. The Party leaders have complete control of all media at all levels, and central, provincial, and city governments to the lowest level, such as factories and villages. The Party's leaders' will is the so-called 'party line', and this is the main message disseminated through television, newspapers, and popular magazines. These official voices are transmitted to every individual in society and reinforced through two main channels: the public media and the Party's internal hierarchy organizations, which consist of all levels of the Communist Party committees. At all of these levels, the Party committees, from central government to neighbourhood Party committees, are the means used to carry out control, and ensure that people conform to the party line. This controlling machine is powered by fear. Every Party committee, from central to local level, is responsible for the territory it covers. If an incident occurs that is outside the party line, the Party leader in charge will be punished. The party line has been the 'life-line' for Chinese people because it controls all aspects of their lives and possibly the survival of entire families, from promotions, privileges, jobs, education, food supply, bonuses and housing to childbirth. Acting outside of the party line means being cut out of everything mentioned above; what is worse, it means labour camps, gaols, and even the death penalty.

Chinese people have learned hard lessons throughout recurrent political movements during the past 53 years of Communist rule, including the destructive 10 years of the Cultural Revolution. Whoever opposes, or just has an opinion that differs from, the party line is in immediate danger. People have learned that it is better to accept the propaganda, since independent thinking and belief are unsafe. In the past two decades, while China has advanced in the economic arena, the Party has appeared to lose some political control, partially due to private companies having some autonomy. However, the massive, brutal persecution of Falun Gong over the past two-plus years, which affects millions of peaceful citizens, including those who work for private companies, has proved that the Party's tight political control is very much alive and well, just as it was in the past. The elements of a modern free market economy introduced into China only distract attention from, and obscure, this political control. What the Communist Party fears most is losing control of people's hearts and minds, and so its control of what people believe is especially tight.

This social and mind control plays an important role in the suppression of millions of Chinese citizens who practise Falun Gong and others whose beliefs are different from Communist ideology. This suppressive social environment has caused millions to live in fear, and poses great danger to their mental health.

Since 5 March 2002, a crisis has been unfolding in the northeastern Chinese city of Changchun, where virtual martial law has been imposed. Police have arrested more than 5,000 'suspected' Falun Gong practitioners since 5 March. Some residents reported screams of torture in the night outside Changchun police stations. Others tell of those who have been beaten to death in police custody. Multiple eyewitnesses describe individuals being thrown from high-rise buildings. Sources attest to dozens of deaths and immediate cremations, possibly as many as 100 or more. The scraps of information these reports piece together paint an ominous picture. On 15 March, Amnesty International issued an Urgent Action request for Falun

Gong practitioners in Changchun City:

> Amnesty International believes they are at serious risk of torture or ill-treatment ... police 'stop and search' checkpoints have reportedly been established across the city ...
>
> (Falun Dafa Information Center, 2002d)

Propaganda and hate campaign

The aim of the Chinese government's campaign has been to control people's minds and to seed hate against Falun Gong in order to carry out and sustain this brutal and unprecedented violation of human rights. Massive government funds have been spent saturating television and radio programmes and print media with lies. This propaganda is not limited to China but has extended overseas to international governments, officials (Rosett, 2002), media (Falun Dafa Information Center, 2000a, 2000b), organizations and individuals. Immediately after the ban, the Chinese television network (which is owned and operated by the government) began to broadcast vicious propaganda against Falun Gong several times every hour. On television, the Chinese people have been shown, over and over again, fabricated cases about people allegedly dying because of Falun Gong. The propaganda completely disregards the health improvement of millions, including those cured of terminal illnesses, and instead has invented the fiction of 1,400 cases of people said to have died from practising Falun Gong. Despite the Chinese government's recent claims, however, there is simply no supporting evidence that Falun Gong can cause harm. The 'evidence' the government has provided is highly suspicious: several cases of so-called 'Falun Gong-induced deaths' that have been independently investigated have proved to be fictitious (Falun Dafa, Minghui, 2001). In addition, suicides, homicides, and other crimes have been falsely blamed on Falun Gong.

Another tactic has been to claim that Falun Gong causes mental illness by falsely labelling those with pre-existing mental illness as Falun Gong practitioners. Several murder cases have been used in the propaganda, such as the Fu case, which was broadcast particularly widely. During a psychotic episode in November 2001, Fu killed his father and wife and severely injured his mother. Sadly, he still seemed to be psychotic during the interview that took place on 17 December 2001 (Galli, 2002). He was not only delusional, but also having command hallucinations. A family member of Fu told his colleague (Ma Ruijin) that eight years ago Fu used to run in the street naked and the family could not control him. It seems that he has a long history of mental illness with violent episodes (Falun Dafa, Clearwisdom, 2002b). The government had used the sad story of Fu's mental illness to frame Falun Gong.

Most of the people used in the propaganda have a long history of severe mental illness and there has been no proof that they were Falun Gong practitioners. In some cases, people had learned some of the exercises on their own, but this does not make them practitioners, as they are not following the basic principles of Falun Gong. A useful analogy would be for someone who received medical treatment for terminal cancer. It would be ridiculous to say that it was the medications he was taking that caused him to die rather than his terminal illness. In the Fu case and other suicide/homicide cases, the real cause of such violence was the individual's long-standing mental illness. There is no foundation for attributing the insane acts of murder to Falun Gong.

Despite government attempts to distort the truth to frame Falun Gong, the content of this politically motivated propaganda is very weak. Chinese official media reports of these fabricated or distorted cases usually do not include psychiatric or forensic examination, nor medical examination, and no (or very few) interviews with family, neighbours or co-workers, except for short answers that parrot the official party line. No independent or international investigations are allowed. The question remains: 'Why have there been no reports of similar outbreaks of mental and physical illness occurring among the numerous overseas Falun Gong communities in recent years?' (Munro, 2002). Furthermore, no suicide or homicide cases were ever reported among the hundreds of thousands of people practising Falun Gong in China before the persecution began, or in 50 countries outside China.

The Chinese government went so far as to stage an event of self-immolation of five individuals in Tiananmen Square on 23 January 2001. They used this to justify the escalation of the persecution, to turn public opinion against Falun Gong, and to further defame the founder, Li Hongzhi, internationally. A week after the incident, the Chinese government television network, CCTV, broadcast a programme showing film of the incident, but in the film the number of victims was increased from five to seven (Falun Information Center, 2001a). Several Chinese state-run newspapers said that the close-up shots in the video were taken from the videotape confiscated from CNN, but the CNN cameras were actually confiscated before the incident unfolded. In the programme, CCTV also broadcast the heartbreaking pictures of 12-year-old Liu Siying, who was severely burned. The propaganda also showed her mother, Liu Chunling, dying from self-immolation, but when the videotape made by the government itself is played in slow motion, it is very clear that Liu Chunling collapsed not from the flames but from being bludgeoned by a man in a military overcoat. Falun Gong members identified the man as a police officer (Radin, 2001). The government intensified the campaign against Falun Gong by forcing every citizen to sign a form condemning Falun Gong, using the pictures of Liu

Siying to foment the public's hatred towards Falun Gong. Western media were sceptical. The *Washington Post*, after some investigative reporting, released a story questioning whether some of the burned victims were in actuality associated with Falun Gong. The journalist went to Liu's home town and asked many of Liu's neighbours. 'There was something wrong with her,' said her neighbour Liu Min, 'No one ever saw her practise Falun Gong' (Pan, 2001). A non-governmental organization (NGO) stated at the United Nations in its August 2001 report:

> The regime points to a supposed self-immolation incident in Tiananmen Square on January 23, 2001, as proof that Falun Gong is an 'evil cult'. However, we have obtained a video of that incident that in our view proves that this event was staged by the government.
> (International Education Development's Statement at the UN [Excerpt]
> Sub-Commission on the Promotion and Protection of
> Human Rights, Fifty-third session, August 2001)

This is just an example of how far the government is willing to go to deceive and manipulate both the international media and people's minds. The cases are too numerous to be mentioned. Sources inside China stated that the order coming from the top is to label as suicide any Falun Gong practitioner's death due to torture. This way suicide becomes both the ticket to kill and the official cover-up for these deaths.

Despite the propaganda being so unreasonable and lacking in credibility, the government is able to continue this deception because their massive brainwashing campaign uses all means of diffusion and control. For example, in schools, children are forced to recite a poem attacking Falun Gong, and have to answer ('correctly') exam questions about Falun Gong. Students at all levels, employees in factories, hospitals, government bureaux and private companies, passengers wanting to take buses and trains, people passing through travel checkpoints, and even individuals walking on the streets, are all forced verbally to support the Communist Party's persecution, step on photos of Li Hongzhi, or denounce or swear against Falun Gong. They must do so in order to get their travel tickets, passports, documents, or benefits such as pensions or health care. If they do not, they are detained and subjected to interrogation and mistreatment.

The blockage of information

The information embargo is an important key in the campaign against Falun Gong that enables Jiang's regime to build up and sustain such brutality. The government censors all coverage by the international media of the persecution in all Chinese television networks and newspapers, and blocks access on the Internet to this information. E-mails and phone calls are monitored. People are arrested just for visiting Falun Gong websites in China. Falun Gong practitioners are detained, sentenced to labour camp or gaol for passing flyers or other material revealing the truth about human rights violations. Tens of millions of Falun Gong books have been confiscated and burned, along with audio and video tapes. All Falun Gong materials have been banned. As a result, the Chinese people do not have access to the truth and do not have any way of knowing that the accusations made by the government are false. This information blackout, the lies, and the fabricated accusations are poisoning the minds of millions of Chinese people, while the 610 office has ordered and orchestrated detentions, sentences to labour camp, rapes, psychiatric abuse, and torture and deaths that proceed silently, unnoticed by the world.

However, in fear of the truth being revealed and the lies and cover-up being exposed, the Chinese government uses extreme measures to block any investigations. These include threatening or bribing family members, immediate cremation of the victims' bodies without forensic examination, and detaining anybody who knows the true story or who tries to reveal the truth to Western media, while censoring the Internet and restricting the access of international media (Falun Dafa Information Center, 2001b; Tsukimori, 2001).

The Chinese Court sentenced US green card holder Teng Chunyan, a 37-year-old acupuncturist from New York, to three years in prison in December 2000. She was accused of spying because she exposed the detention of Falun Gong practitioners in mental hospitals to the Western media (Agence France Presse, 2000).

China has also blocked attempts at investigation by international organizations such as Amnesty International. Meanwhile, in the past year, many foreign journalists who have attempted to investigate these matters (or, in some cases, merely cover Falun Gong) have been detained, harassed, had their licences revoked, and in some cases even been deported from China (Donohoe, 2001; Johnson, 2000b; Restall, 2001).

Brainwashing

The Chinese government uses every torture technique learned through China's long history, and much more. Presently, they have hundreds of brainwashing centres throughout the country with the specific purpose of forcing Falun Gong practitioners to denounce and give up the practice. Practitioners are brought to these centres by force, sometimes after being kidnapped off the street or from their workplaces or homes.

Near the Wuchang No. 2 Bridge on the Changjiang River is a prison holding approximately 40 Falun Gong practitioners. This is the Wuchang 610 office's brainwashing class, which officials from the Wuchang District of Wuhan City, Hubei Province, have created specifically to torture Falun Gong practitioners. Carrying out Jiang's orders, the brainwashing class employs a team of 'brainwashing specialists' who actively persecute those practitioners who remain steadfast in their belief. In the past years, countless Falun Gong practitioners have been illegally detained and persecuted here. Furthermore, determined practitioners who have completed their detention terms in forced labour camps and still refuse to stop practising Falun Gong are sent to this brainwashing class for persecution (Falun Dafa Information Center, 2002b). The Wuchang 610 office has received many 'awards' from the provincial and city governments for its 'achievements' in persecuting Falun Gong. Many delegates from other regions come and learn from their experience of how to coerce agreement with torture. Another well-known place of torture is Masanjia Labour Camp, where practitioners are not only being tortured but also performing forced labour. The brainwashing classes totally violate the country's constitution and laws by holding Dafa practitioners in detention for an unlimited period of time without cause.

The cruelty of the methods used is beyond description. They have set up so-called 'brainwashing classes' where practitioners are forced to watch, for hours on end, films that slander Falun Dafa. Full of lies and fabrications, these films are meant to convince the practitioners to stop the practice. The classes are used in conjunction with sleep deprivation and other tortures, both mental and physical. Practitioners are kept awake for days, and endure all kinds of torture, including rape. At times a number of gaolers scream at them if they fall asleep, insulting them and cursing Falun Gong and Li Hongzhi. They are kept in small, dark, damp, rat-infested individual cells. Practitioners are kept handcuffed with their hands behind their backs in a fixed position that does not allow them to move or lie down. The basin provided in the cell must be used for both washing and for defecation and urination. Sometimes the handcuffs are fastened to the ground, forcing prisoners to sit on the ground or to crawl. Wardens punish them by forcing them to squat for long periods tying them in painful body contortions, or applying electric shocks. The torture is only stopped if they sign a letter defaming Falun Dafa and promising to stop the practice. Some bodies are tortured beyond recognition. A brutal and slow death comes to those who refuse to renounce their belief.

Many previous mentally healthy Falun Gong practitioners, including scientists, became insane after severe torture beyond the limits of human endurance. Lin Chengtao was a graduate from the Chinese Academy of Medical Sciences and Peking Union Medical College, where he proved to be a brilliant medical scientist and a key person in his research group. His mind was destroyed and he can no longer take care of himself. He has been in the notorious Tuanhe Labour Camp since September 2001. Lin has refused to give up the practice of Falun Gong. Thrown into solitary confinement, the guards tortured Lin daily with electric shock clubs that have a charge of 30,000 volts. This torture eventually took Lin's sanity. Incredibly, even though he has lost his mind, the guards there continue to torture him daily. Whereas before they tortured him for practising Falun Gong, now they torture him because they say he is faking mental illness (Falun Dafa, Minghui, 2002).

Abuse of psychiatry

Once one comes to know of the campaign of terror that has been waged by the Chinese government since July 1999, the extensive abuse of psychiatry as another form of persecution and mind control comes as no surprise. Under orders from the police, psychiatric and medical personnel torture healthy detainees with high doses of anti-psychotic medications, high voltage electric shocks and other methods of torture to carry out the orders of the Chinese Communist Party.

Ninety psychiatric institutions have been documented as engaging in this kind of abuse (Falun Dafa Information Center, 2002e). In addition, even more brutal tortures are taking place in at least 20 *Ankang* [peace and health] (Munro, 2001) institutions, owned by the Ministry of Public Security. The length of detention has ranged from seven days to over two years. Torture has left many victims both physically and mentally disabled. Several have died while in detention or shortly after being discharged from the hospitals. Today the number of normal, healthy practitioners who have been incarcerated in mental health hospitals far exceeds 1,000.

From the outset of the Chinese regime's persecution of Falun Gong and as early as September 1999, the police have forced practitioners to be incarcerated in mental health facilities without cause. The government then uses police to control psychiatric facilities in an effort to coerce practitioners to renounce their beliefs. Many reports from inside China indicate that practitioners who continue to express conviction in their spiritual practice are illegally injected with sedatives, anti-psychotics and nerve-damaging drugs. Other abuse in the mental hospitals includes both physical and mental torture. The following two cases are examples.

Su Gang was a 32-year-old computer engineer working at the Qi-Lu Oil Chemical Company. He was repeatedly detained by the security department of his workplace for refusing to renounce Falun Gong. His family has stated that Su Gang was in good health and had no mental illness prior to his detention. The *Washington Post* reported:

> After traveling to Beijing on April 25 to protest the ban on Falun Gong, he was arrested again; on May 23, his employer, a state-run petrochemical company, approved commitment papers that authorized the police to admit him

to a mental hospital. According to Mr. Su's father, the doctors injected Mr. Su twice a day with an unknown substance. When Mr. Su emerged a week later, he could not eat or move his limbs normally.

(*Washington Post*, 2000)

Nor could he remember what happened to him in the hospital; he even stopped speaking. On 10 June the previously healthy young man died (Falun Dafa, Clearwisdom, 2000a; Su and Su, 2000).

Shi Bei was a 49-year-old woman who had no history of mental illness. She was involuntarily admitted to Hangzhou Mental Health Hospital. She was administered unknown substances and was later starved to death. Officials from the hospital refused to comment to the reporter (Falun Dafa, Clearwisdom, 2000b, 2000c).

Perphenazine, chlorpromazine, fluphenazine, fluorohydroxypiperidine and other, unknown, substances are frequently administered by force-feeding patients or mixing drugs into their food. As a result, many practitioners suffer severe toxic effects such as loss of memory, severe headaches, fainting, extreme weakness, uncontrollable tremors, nausea, vomiting, seizures, and loss of consciousness. Some severe cases resemble neuroleptic malignant syndrome. Medications are delivered at many times the therapeutic dose and thus often result in devastating and irreversible consequences (Lu and Galli, 2002). Tying individuals to beds and force-feeding medications through nasogastric tubing, handcuffing or tying patients up in very painful postures for long periods of time, burning detainees' skin with electric batons, insertion of acupuncture needles deep into the muscles, and applying electric current to produce excruciating pain have all been added to a long list of cruel and abusive tactics of mind control.

Doctors have made clear statements indicating that Falun Gong practitioners are admitted, not in relation to their health, but for political reasons. 'The doctors told him they knew he was sane but were under orders from their superiors in the police department to "treat" him anyway' (Pan, 2002.) Some medical staff even taunt practitioners, saying such things as, 'Aren't you practising Falun Gong? Let's see which is stronger, Falun Gong or our medicines' (Falun Dafa, Clearwisdom, 2000d). One nurse reportedly stated: 'This is the way to persecute ... [your] religion.' This cruel battle that pits the hospital staff against the sanity and the life of the practitioners only ends when the practitioners meet the criteria for discharge, i.e. only when they stop performing Falun Gong exercises, and sign a pledge to renounce their belief in Falun Gong. In the more unfortunate cases, some practitioners were discharged because they were dying from abuse. Some psychiatric hospitals rate themselves as being successful in converting Falun Gong practitioners. It is a sad truth that many hospitals in China can now be listed along with state prisons and forced labour camps as government facilities for persecution and torture.

In 1991, the United Nations established *Principles for the Protection of Persons with Mental Illness* and for the *Improvement of Mental Health Care*. According to Principle 4 of this important UN document: 'A determination that a person has a mental illness shall be made in accordance with internationally accepted medical standards. A determination of mental illness shall never be made on the basis of political, economic or social status or membership in a cultural, racial or religious group, or for any other reason not directly relevant to mental health status.' Principle 10 states: 'Medication shall meet the best health needs of the patient, shall be given to a patient only for therapeutic or diagnostic purposes and shall never be administered as a punishment or for the convenience of others' (United Nations, 1991). China's growth of appalling psychiatric abuse violates all patient rights stated in the United Nations Declaration of Human Rights Assembly 1948, to which China is a signatory.

The American Psychiatric Association (APA) and the Royal College of Psychiatry have played an important role in alerting international psychiatric organizations of the ongoing abuse of psychiatry in China. In April 2000 members of the APA presented the news of the persecution of Falun Gong practitioners in mental hospitals, during the second Sino-American Psychiatric Conference in Beijing. During the APA annual meeting in Chicago 2000, the Committee on Misuse and Abuse of Psychiatry requested the Board of Trustees to endorse their petition for a request for an investigation by the World Psychiatric Association (WPA). By summer 2000, Borenstein, the APA president, contacted the WPA to inform them of the psychiatric abuse in China and to request an investigation. In April 2001, the Geneva Initiative on Psychiatry released a press statement condemning the abuse of Falun Gong practitioners and called for an investigation. The Royal College of Psychiatry, during the General Meeting in London, July 2001, unanimously passed a resolution to send a team of international experts to investigate abuse of psychiatry in China. During that meeting the WPA president elect, Ahmed Okasha expressed the WPA's concern for the psychiatric abuse of Falun Gong practitioners in China. In Madrid, August 2001, the WPA presented a symposium on the abuse of psychiatry in China, and Marianne Kastrup, chairwoman of the WPA review committee, reported progress on the response of the Chinese Psychiatric Association.

In May 2001, in New Orleans, during the APA Annual Meeting, the Commission on Global Psychiatry and the Committee of Misuse and Abuse of Psychiatry reviewed the six known cases of death as a consequence of psychiatric abuse and the progress of the WPA's upcoming investigation. An Action Paper condemning the Chinese government's misuse of psychiatry was initiated by Nicholas Stratas and Peggy Dorfman and was unanimously passed by the APA General Assembly, urging the WPA to act on the ongoing abuses of psychiatry. Lopez Ibor met with the Minister of Health in China to discuss the abuses of psychiatry and requested an internal investigation.

In Philadelphia in May 2002, Abraham Halpern, an APA human rights award recipient in 2001, spoke of the use of long-acting high doses of neuroleptic medications on Falun Gong practitioners by Chinese medical staff. On 20 May, Lifers (life members of the APA) unanimously supported the motion for the APA to persuade the WPA to move with the investigation without further delay. The WPA held a symposium on patients' rights and informed consent, where the purpose and meaning of informed consent was defined as a 'moral contract'. Lopez Ibor, president of the WPA, spoke of the need for psychiatrists to adhere to the Madrid Declaration and warned against the use of psychiatry for political purposes.

Finally, during the WPA Psychiatric Congress held in August 2002, Yokohama, Japan, the general assembly, composed of member societies from 120 countries, passed a resolution to proceed with an independent investigation of psychiatric abuse in China as a means for the persecution of Falun Gong practitioners. The WPA stated that they would like to initiate this investigation some time in the autumn of 2002 and to have a report available for the APA annual meeting in spring 2003. Lopez Ibor announced the willingness of the Chinese authorities to allow an international team of experts to visit mental health hospitals.

The past three years of peaceful appeals by Falun Gong practitioners inside and outside China have achieved remarkable results, breaking through the information blockade. International organizations and governments have responded to the persecution by publicly condemning these severe human rights violations (Amnesty International, 2001; Freedom House, 2001; Jendrzejczyk and Spiegel, 1999). On 24 July 2002, the US House of Representatives unanimously passed Resolution 188, stating:

> Resolved by the House of Representatives (the Senate concurring), that it is the sense of Congress that
>
> 1. the Government of the People's Republic of China should cease its persecution of Falun Gong practitioners, and its representatives in the United States should cease their harassment of citizens and residents of the United States who practice Falun Gong and cease their attempts to put pressure on officials of State and local governments in the United States to refuse or withdraw support for the Falun Gong and its practitioners;
> 2. the United States Government should use every appropriate public and private forum to urge the Government of the People's Republic of China –
>   (a) to release from detention all Falun Gong practitioners and put an end to the practices of torture and other cruel, inhumane, and degrading treatment against them and other prisoners of conscience; and (b) to abide by

the International Covenant on Civil and Political Rights and the Universal Declaration of Human Rights by allowing Falun Gong practitioners to pursue their personal beliefs; and ...

(United States Congress, 2002)

Despite over half a century of Communist Party suppression on 1.3 billion Chinese citizens, the present tight mind control and blockage of information are doomed to fail in today's era of modern global economy and information. Moreover, the spread from China of severe acute respiratory syndrome (SARS) has vividly revealed the danger of such a policy to both Chinese citizens and the world. Facing harsh treatment such as imprisonment, torture and even death, millions of courageous Falun Gong practitioners have come forward to reveal the truth of this horrible persecution to the international community through the Internet and other communication channels. The voice of justice condemning the persecution arises from all around the world. With international pressure that objects to the massive, systematic abuse of human rights, China will begin to honour the freedoms of conscience, belief and expression, the most fundamental of human rights. We must act now to help stop the killing of Falun Gong practitioners. We must not remain silent.

References

Agence France Presse (2000) China Charges US Resident with Spying for Exposing Falun Gong Crackdown. Agence France Press, 23 Nov. http://www.clearwisdom.net/emh/articles/2000/11/25/6029.html.

Amnesty International (2001) Torture – A Growing Scourge in China. Time for Action (Excerpts). ASA. 17 April.

Donohoe M (2001) Censors have their work cut out in press-shy China. Irish Times, 25 June: 13.

Falun Dafa (2002) What is Falun Gong? www.FalunDafa.org.

Falun Dafa, Clearwisdom (2000a) The Truth Behind the Death of Mr. Su Gang. 21 June. http://www.clearwisdom.net/emh/articles/2000/6/21/8769.html.

Falun Dafa, Clearwisdom (2000b) My Mother was Starved to Death by Police for Practicing Falun Gong. 30 September. http://www.clearwisdom.net/emh/articles/2000/9/30/8097.html.

Falun Dafa, Clearwisdom (2000c) Press Statement from Practitioners in Canada. 1 October. http://www.clearwisdom.net/emh/articles/2000/10/1/6660.html.

Falun Dafa, Clearwisdom (2000d) Practitioner Detained and Forced to Take Injections in Mental Hospital for more than Two Months. 8 February. http://www.clearwisdom.net/emh/articles/2000/2/8/8620.html.

Falun Dafa, Clearwisdom (2002a) Governmental Awards and Recognition of Falun Dafa from China and the World, 2002. http://www.clearwisdom.net/emh/special_column/recognition.html.

Falun Dafa, Clearwisdom (2002b) 'Capital Murder Case's' Fu Yibin was Insane According to Relative. 2 February. http://www.clearwisdom.net/emh/articles/2002/2/2/18336.html

Falun Dafa Information Center (2000a) A Look at Jiang's Attack on Hong Kong Journalists. 17 November. http://faluninfo.net/displayAnArticle.asp?ID=1247

Falun Dafa Information Center (2000b) Jiang Zemin's Representatives Attempt to Control the Australian Media. 5 December. http://faluninfo.net/displayAnArticle.asp?ID=1523

Falun Dafa Information Center (2001a) A Staged Tragedy – Was the So-called 'Self-immolation' a Setup? January. http://www.faluninfo.net/tiananmen/immolation.asp

Falun Dafa Information Center (2001b) Monitoring News of the Persecution of Falun Gong. China Crisis News Bulletin, 87: 1.

Falun Dafa Information Center (2002a) Jiang Zemin Orders 'Kill Them Without Mercy' After Surprise TV Broadcast in China Supports Falun Gong, 7 March. http://www.faluninfo.net/DisplayAnArticle.asp?ID=5397

Falun Dafa Information Center (2002b) Front Page. http://www.faluninfo.net

Falun Dafa Information Center (2002c) 610: An Overview. http://www.faluninfo.net/devstories/610/index.asp

Falun Dafa Information Center (2002d) A Crisis Unfolds in Changchun. 2 April. http://www.faluninfo.net/DisplayAnArticle.asp?ID=5509

Falun Dafa Information Center (2002e) Psychiatric Abuses Report. August. http://www.faluninfo.net/hrreports/PsychAbuse.pdf

Falun Dafa, Minghui (2001) A Question to Beijing TV Station: The Truth About 1400 Death Cases. 26 January. http://package.minghui.org/zhenxiang_ziliao/ziliao_huibian/fake_report/2_13.html

Falun Dafa, Minghui (2002) Four Dafa Practitioners Suffer Mental Breakdowns Due to Severe Torture at Tuanhe Labor Camp, Beijing. 13 July. http://www.minghui.org/mh/articles/2002/7/2/32691.html

Fang B (1999) An Opiate of the Masses. U.S. News and World Report. 22 February.

Freedom House (2001) Freedom House's Speech at 57th Session of the UN Commission on Human Rights. 11 April. http://www.clearwisdom.net/emh/articles/2001/4/11/7001.html

Galli V (2002) An American Psychiatrist's Comments: The Fu Yibin Case is a Psychiatric Case. 17 January. http://www.clearwisdom.net/emh/articles/2002/1/17/17862.html

United States Congress (2002) House of Representatives Resolution 188. United States Congress, 24 July.

He Mai (2002) Pooled Analysis of Falun Gong Health Effect Survey. Proceeding of 1st World Congress of Future Science and Culture V (001): 3. http://www.zhengjian.org/zj/articles/2002/3/11/14055.html

International Education Development (IED) (2001) Statement at the United Nations Sub-Commission on the Promotion and Protection of Human Rights, 53rd session, Agenda item 6, August: 1. http://www.clearwisdom.net/emh/articles/2001/10/20/14900.html

Jendrzejczyk M, Spiegel M (1999) United Nations must Censure China for Rights Violations. Human Rights Watch. 27 December.

Johnson I (2000a) A deadly exercise. Practicing Falun Gong was a right Ms. Chen said, to her last day. Wall Street Journal, 20 April: A1.

Johnson I. (2000b) A Daughter in China Follows Tortuous Path to Seek Justice. Wall Street Journal, 2 October: A1.

Lu S, Galli V (2002) Psychiatric Abuse of Falun Gong Practitioners in China. Journal of the Academy of Psychiatry and the Law, 30: 26–30.

Munro R (2001) AWSJ Column: China's Judicial Psychiatry. 2 February. http://faluninfo.net/displayAnArticle.asp?ID=3444

Munro R (2002) Dangerous Minds. Human Rights Watch. Geneva Initiative On Psychiatry, pp.172–3.

Pan PP (2001) Human Fire Ignites Chinese Mystery; Motive for Public Burning Intensifies Fight over Falun Gong. Washington Post, 4 February.

Pan PP (2002) The Silent Treatment from Beijing. Mental Hospitals Allegedly Used to Quiet Dissidents, Falun Gong. Washington Post, 26 August: A01. http://www.washingtonpost.com/wp-dyn/articles/A60968-2002Aug25.html

Radin CA (2001) Falun Gong Appeals for Help. Boston Globe, 18 April.

Restall H (2001) Don't Gamble the Olympics on Beijing. Asian Wall Street Journal, 4 July: 17.

Rosett C (2002) Will Chinese Repression Play in Peoria? Beijing's campaign against an 'evil cult' comes to America. Wall Street Journal, 21 February.

Su Y, Su LX (2000) The Open Letter from Mr. Su Gang's Family Members to the Authority, 21 June. http://www.clearwisdom.net/emh/articles/2000/6/21/8770.html

Tsukimori O (2001) Falun Gong asks Bush for help. Washington Times, 8 September: A5.

United Nations (1991) Principles for the Protection of Persons with Mental Illness and for the Improvement of Mental Health Care. New York: United Nations.

Washington Post (2000) Editorial, Bad Medicine in China. 22 June. http://www.washingtonpost.com/wp-dyn/articles/A45724-2000Jun22.html

Wo-Lap Lam W (2001) China's suppression carries a high price. 6 February. CNN, 11:7.

CHAPTER TEN

Mental health in a post-war society: A history of neglect and denial of medical pluralism in Mozambique

VICTOR IGREJA

Introduction

After colonialism, internal armed conflicts, failed Marxist–Leninist policies, systems of injustice and impunity, corruption, and poverty, the professional mental health care sector in Mozambique remains a marginal priority and a privilege confined to a minority of urban citizens. The majority of rural people are precluded from professional assistance. Family networks, traditional medicine and religious groups are the main resources available to address mental health problems of both rural and urban citizens. The extent that these resources effectively help patients with mental health problems to overcome their condition is not well known. However, there are at least two important factors that play a key role in understanding the present 'state of the art' of the mental health sector in Mozambique.

First, medical pluralism has a long history of denial and political persecution, which began with the former Portuguese colonizers and, paradoxically, continued intensively after independence in 1975. Second, 16 years of civil war, interposed by natural disasters that severely affected the majority of the poor and rural population, only recently triggered the empathy of governmental and non-governmental organizations (both national and international) to develop programmes to address psychosocial suffering of trauma survivors (WHO, 1997, 2000). Despite these programmes and initiatives, there is a huge gap between the immensity of mental problems and the local capabilities both in terms of human and financial resources to respond.

The field of professional mental health care has few available reports discussing the nature of mental health policies and practices in Mozambique post-independence (Mandlhate, 1996). Nor are there epidemiological studies to estimate the prevalence of mental health problems. Very little is known about the potential contributions of traditional medicine and religious groups to treating mental disturbances of both rural and urban citizens throughout the country (Green, 1996). However, it is generally recognized that traditional healers and religious leaders play an underestimated role in the provision of health care in Mozambique. Gradually the healers' work is being recognized by the Mozambican official authorities while professional mental health care remains a human right serving only some urban elite. This chapter focuses on the key features of the mental health sector in Mozambique, that is, the historical process, post-colonial policies and strategies applied by the government and non-governmental organizations to respond to the mental health problems resulting from prolonged and multiple exposure to trauma. Emphasis is given to the irreconcilable contradictions of using Western-inspired categorizations of mental health and distress in a non-Western and medical pluralistic society. To illustrate this observation a community-based research study conducted in the former war zones of central Mozambique is used.

Historical background

Mental health: A history of marginality

Interest in the mental health sector, combined with the vital need to recognize and invest in local cultural resources to address problems of mental health, has a short history in Mozambique's post-colonial period. It appears that, historically, the dominant discourse – implicit or explicit – is that mental health problems are a rare phenomenon among people throughout the African continent (German, 1987). The lack of national policies, allied to the lack of skilled human resources and inadequate infrastructure and essential psychotropic drugs, shapes the present condition of individuals and families suffering from mental problems (Bondestam, 1994).

There are several reasons in Mozambique for the continuous process of neglect of the mental health sector. First, the organizational system of mental health services was inherited from the Portuguese Colonial Administration. It was primarily conceived to respond to the mental health problems of the Portuguese citizens living in Mozambique until the date of independence, and not for the majority of Mozambican patients. To disrupt even more the availability and accessibility of mental health care, the Portuguese administration forbade the practice of traditional medicine in Mozambique. The right of medical pluralism that shapes the therapeutic choices of patients and their families was denied, and traditional healers had to work on the edges of the rigid colonial administration.

Second, after Mozambique's independence, the majority of Portuguese mental health professionals departed the country and there were no Mozambican specialist professionals available to respond to the urgent demand characteristic of the transitional phase from violent colonialism to disruptive and degenerative Marxist–Leninist policies. To fill the gap, the Mozambican state relied on the co-operation of Marxist countries, and some mental health professionals, mainly from Cuba and the former Soviet Union, began working in the few psychiatric institutions left by the Portuguese settlers. The interventions of the 'new' psychiatrists loaded with revolutionary knowledge were mainly curative.

Third, in the post-colonial period, the mental health care sector was not considered a priority and did not exist even as a subsystem of the national health care system.[1] The majority of public investment in health was concentrated on primary health care which precluded mental health care services. The same tendency is evident today. Barely a sentence can be found referring to mental health in the country in any of the annual reports from the Ministry of Health or from the United Nations Development Programme (1999).

Fourth, the Mozambican state neither respected nor tried to invest in local cultural practices as part of available resources to deal with mental health problems. On the contrary, the traditional system of beliefs and practices of community organizations did not match with Marxist–Leninist ideology, which shaped the convictions of the Mozambican politicians in the years following independence. As a result, traditional and religious healers were banned, persecuted, accused of threatening the process of state/nation building,[2] and some of them were sent to re-education camps. The healers' crafts and important symbols of their healing 'machinery' were burned in public and their actions were considered blasphemy in the light of the new national order. As one of my informants in Gorongosa district described, his experiences of persecution had two phases. 'At the beginning, we had to resist the Portuguese settlers until the date of independence. We thought that the situation would get better with independence. But to our surprise, Frelimo members began to persecute us like never before. They began to act worse than the Portuguese settlers did. They [Frelimo members] treated us as if we were enemies. They called us "Enemies of the People".'

---

[1] Interview with Dr. Custódia Mandlhate. Dr. Custódia Mandlhate was 1st National Director of the 1st National Mental Health Programme in Mozambique. Currently she is the Regional Advisor for Mental Health and Prevention of Substance Abuse, based in Harare, WHO-AFRO. 23 March 2000, World Health Organization office, Maputo, Mozambique.

[2] This construction was also extended to what was termed 'Formation of the New Man'. The formation was bestowed to the educational system, the media, and to a great extent to the public speeches of the first president of the former Popular Republic of Mozambique, Samora Machel.

These facts have continuously shaped the development of the mental health sector during the last three decades. The state systematically failed to recognize the importance of mental health and to provide financial investment. And to aggravate the situation even more there was a rejection of medical pluralism, and denial of the importance of traditional and religious healers to improve the mental health of the people. According to Custódia Mandlhate, 'Until 1996 the mental health sector was confined to simple curative practices in the two main psychiatric hospitals (Hopistal Psiquiatrico do Infulene in Maputo province and the Hospital Psiquiatrico de Nampula in Nampula province, in the northern region of Mozambique) and different yards that had been left by the colonial administration. There was no such programme that we now designate the National Mental Health Programme.'

War suffering, political reforms and the first National Mental Health Programme

In the mid-1980s the civil war had spread throughout the country and concerns were raised regarding its effects on the well-being of exposed and affected children. The Mozambican government, in partnership with international mental health professionals, conceived a mental health programme to assist the children living in war-affected areas. The programme was designated *Atendimento da criança em situação difícil* [Caring for children in difficult situations].[3] This programme was aimed at caring for the children living in war zones. The strategy adopted was to provide training courses for primary schoolteachers working in these areas on how to identify children with learning, psychological and emotional problems as a result of their exposure to violence. According to Ratilal, at this stage, 'The use of cultural resources such as traditional healers and religious leaders was neither considered nor integrated in this programme because the traditional healers were not yet recognized by the governmental authorities and we knew very little about their work.'

In 1984, the Ministry of Health organized the first national seminar on mental health, and provided basic recommendations for the National Mental Health Programme. The programme was an attempt to give a response to the growing mental health needs of the war-affected population and to follow up the programmes that had been conceived to assist children and their war-traumatized parents. In 1990, the Mozambican state adopted political and economic reforms that ended with the adoption of a

---

[3]   In the absence of a mental health sector in the country, the Ministry of Education and Culture carried out this programme, and it was implemented by the Department of Special Education. Dr. Anabela Ratilal, Director of Centro de Reabilitação Psicologica Infantil e Juvenil [Psychological Rehabilitation Centre for Infants and Youth], Maputo Central Hospital. Dr. Ratilal took part in this programme as a training technician between 1988 and 1991. Interview, 19 April 2000, Central Hospital, Maputo.

multiparty constitution. The recognition of political, medical and religious pluralism was guaranteed at least by the constitutional text, and the contribution of traditional practitioners in health care was gradually and publicly encouraged. As a result of the changes to the political organization, traditional healers created, in 1992, the first Mozambican Association of Traditional Practitioners (AMETRAMO).

The first steps towards the recognition of the mental health needs of the victims of war and natural disasters in Mozambique began in fact with the programme mentioned above. These experiences, combined with endorsements of the World Health Organization (WHO), in which the country was already a member, inspired the creation of the first National Mental Health Programme under the leadership of Mandlhate. The priorities of this programme were defined as follows: (1) substance abuse (drugs, alcohol and tobacco); (2) epilepsy; (3) psychosocial effects of war and other catastrophes; (4) infant psychomotor development; (5) infant behavioural disorders; and (6) chronic mental diseases (Mandlhate, 1996). The programme also recommended the establishment of 'A partnership with the traditional medicine sector' because the governmental authorities officially accepted that traditional healers play a role in communities and that the availability, accessibility, and acceptability of the professional health sector was problematic, in particular, in the mental health sector.

The chronic invisibility of the state in the mental health sector

Despite its official status, the National Mental Health Programme is hampered by a lack of human resources and proper financial input from the governmental authorities. Mental health practices are still confined to curative interventions. The programme is limited to managing the reduced budget provided by the government to cover the wages of the professionals. In the best of the cases and in order to escape from anonymity, every year the leadership of the National Mental Health Programme organizes official ceremonies to celebrate the Mental Health World's Day. For instance, in 2001, the Mental Health World's Day was celebrated under the label of 'Mental Health and Work'. Mozambique celebrated by publicly launching a non-governmental association for mentally ill patients. Through such events the programme justifies its presence and reminds everyone of its existence. To date, most of the projects on mental health have been funded by foreign institutions such as the WHO, the United Nations, and foreign governments. The WHO is one of the few international institutions that have been demonstrating an increasing interest in assessing the psychosocial consequences of armed conflicts, and to find culturally congruent therapies to help survivors recover from the long-term effects of trauma exposure (Mandlhate, 1996; WHO, 1997, 2000). Yet the lack of systematic knowledge about cultural practices used both in times of crisis and in the trauma recovery period has been one of the main stumbling blocks for the conception and implementation of culturally sensitive and cost-effective programmes to address the long-term effects of trauma exposure. This has been recognized by several mental health professionals as intrinsic to other post-armed-conflict countries in non-Western societies around the globe (for example, Hiegel, 1994; Marsella et al., 1996).

Interventions by non-government organizations

In recent years, Mozambican and foreign non-governmental organizations (NGOs) have been playing an important role in the provision of mental health services. Most of the local initiatives were shaped by the politics and systems of beliefs of international donors regarding the mental health status of trauma survivors in non-Western societies. According to Mandlhate: 'There was a time that to get solidarity funds for local projects it was an imperative to use concepts of "trauma", "post-traumatic stress", "victims of war" and so on. If the proposals did not contain such terminology it was not possible to get funds from international donors.' In 1996, the Mental Health Section of the Ministry of Health, in partnership with the University of Hamburg, organized in Maputo the first international and scientific congress entitled 'Children, War and Persecution: Rebuilding Hope'. This congress marked the beginning of different research and intervention initiatives in the field of psychotrauma in Mozambique.

As a result of this congress, different NGOs were created with the support of foreign countries and institutions to work in the field of mental health of trauma survivors. Several psychosocial programmes were launched to respond to the mental health needs of survivors of the armed conflicts and natural disasters that have afflicted Mozambique in the last three decades. These organizations include *Reconstruir a Esperança* [Rebuilding Hope], which concerns the psychosocial problems of the former child soldiers and their traumatized families. Using psychoanalytical models inspired by the German schools of psychoanalysis, this organization tries to make sense of the 'world of spirits' presented in the narratives of former child soldiers and their families.[4] The NGO 'Kulaya' looks after the psychosocial problems of traumatized adolescent, youth and adult women victims of domestic violence, sexual abuse and violation. The infant

---

4 However, according to Eufraime Boia, director of Rebuilding Hope, this NGO is going through a process of transformation and adaptation of its programme for the new Mozambican context. There are no more former child soldiers and their main donor Medico International, based in Germany, is shifting its intervention programmes to other areas of the world.

and youth centre designated *Centro de Reabilitação Psicológica Infantil e Juvenil* [Centre for Psychological Rehabilitation of Infants and Youth], affiliated to the Maputo Central Hospital, attends traumatized children and adolescent victims of rape and sexual abuse. However, according to Ratilal, 'Most of these initiatives are located in the southern region of Mozambique, in urban settings, and they are not capable of providing a full response in relation to the level of mental health demands of trauma survivors.'

These initiatives are also complicated by the fact that differences between the providers and users regarding explanatory models of health and illness impair a full and successful implementation of mental health interventions. According to Mandlhate, 'It is known that many people before they look for help in our health facilities, in particular for psychiatric problems, they look for traditional medicine. For this reason, when we conceived the National Mental Health Programme we emphasized this important cultural aspect as one of the basic conditions to community-based intervention programmes in the post-war period and we stressed the need for systematic research in this field.' While the expected co-operation is taking a long time to start, the therapeutic choices for the majority will be divided between the reduced professional health care assistance, and traditional and religious healing practices – but not the best from, nor complementary to, either world.

Trauma survivors from the former war zones of central Mozambique

In Gorongosa District, the former war zones in central Mozambique, the non-governmental organization *Associação Esperança para Todos* [Hope for Everyone] conducted one of the few epidemiological studies in the post-colonial period. The project was aimed at assessing the effects of war on the physical and mental health of the war survivors with particular emphasis on the prevalence of war memories, pathological forms (nightmares) and post-traumatic symptoms. Longitudinal household surveys combined with anthropological techniques (in-depth interviews and participant observation) were conducted in different communities with a cohort of 700 men and women. Baseline assessment was carried out in 1997 (five years after the end of the war in 1992) and follow-up continued until 1999.

The preliminary results demonstrated that the degree of war and drought exposure was very high (Igreja et al., 1999; Schreuder et al., 2001). Ninety-seven per cent of the people lived in the former war zones during the entire period of 16 years of civil war and had experienced more than 15 different traumatic events. The high prevalence of post-traumatic reactions correlated with the high degree of war and drought exposure. People complained of a range of psychological, somatic and sociocultural problems. They complained of sleep disorders and nightmares, intrusive thoughts and memories of traumatic experiences, and avoiding behaviours, including the use of psychoactive substances. Somatic symptoms were also diagnosed, including headache, physical weakness, dizziness, poor appetite, and tiredness.

This study has also drawn four important conclusions. First, it has demonstrated how complicated and ineffective it is to use Western standardized instruments to measure the prevalence and severity of war-related mental health problems among trauma survivors in a non-Western society. Second, people's perceptions of the effects of the war and drought are not linked primarily to psychopathological consequences susceptible to measurement with the scientific rigour of the narrow-minded Western psychiatric academia. Local cultural perceptions and interpretations of the consequences of overwhelming experiences are explained in the first place in terms of the deregulation and disruption of sociocultural, historical and political processes. Third, even with the use of validated standardized instruments, the rigour of measurements or controlled interventions is undermined and critically confronted by the particularities of the production cycle. For instance, there is a high probability that baseline measurements carried out at the onset of the agricultural cycle will yield a different result to the same measurement carried out at the end of the agricultural cycle. Fourth, in the present context of Mozambique, characterized by an overwhelming increase of state-based corruption which aggravates the scenario of poverty and misery, the magnitude and complexity of mental health problems can be better perceived and tackled when applying longitudinal approaches and not through rapid and short-term methodological techniques. Because of the relevance of these findings to the overall understanding of the present situation in the field of mental health in Mozambique, a description of each of the four above points is justified.

Psychiatric instruments

The use of standardized instruments during the Gorongosa study in central Mozambique has confirmed the fact that measuring instruments cannot be universally applied across cultures (Bracken et al., 1995; Eisenbruch, 1991). Several problems were identified. The first is posed by language differences. Our research suggests that it is not always possible to translate psychological concepts into the local language. The problem is further complicated when the local languages are not yet written and specificity of meaning needs to be revealed by repeated translations. These in turn are tested and re-tested using as many local people as possible.

The second challenge is related to the conceptual equivalence of items, scales or measures. For instance, concepts such as 'nervous', 'health', 'disturbed', 'palpitation', and 'unhappy' are extremely difficult concepts to translate accurately in the local language.

The third problem is related to the standardized way in which patients are expected to give their answers to the diagnostic instruments. For example, although there are equivalent translations in the local language to rate items 'not at all' and 'slightly', 'seriously' and 'extremely' are not used in the daily language of the people. This means that the latter two distinctions aimed at assessing the severity of symptoms are inappropriate and irrelevant.

The fourth problem is the time period used to assess the appearance of different symptoms. For example, some questionnaires use length of time, such as 'last or previous four weeks'. In most cases, the people do not manage their daily lives by measuring time in this way. Rather their time is guided by natural phenomena (for example, the different phases or appearance of the moon) or more importantly, the agricultural cycle. So, when someone in the sample is asked, 'Have you had headaches in the last four weeks?' the answer cannot be given – not because the person does not understand the content of the question, but because the length or interval of time does not make sense. A typical construction using the agricultural cycle as a temporal frame of reference to narrate an event can be illustrated by the following example from an interview with a grandmother referring to the timeframe of her granddaughter's tragic death: 'The first rain to start sowing passed [October]. The people began to do sowing [also October]. Then we began weeding until finish [November]. My daughter gave birth and there was no problem. Then the people went on to do the second weeding [December and January]. We started to eat maize [February] and when the maize was starting to get dry [between March and April], the baby suddenly got ill, and she died.' Without acquiring insights into the dynamics of the production cycle this accurate answer could perplex an unfamiliar health professional.

The fifth problem is related to the way people register and interpret traumatic experiences. For instance, contrary to general perception, death of a family member may not be as traumatic an experience as the failure to bury appropriately the body of the deceased. This is because of the negative consequences associated with breaking culturally prescribed rituals. This approach in the manifestation and expression of distress has tremendous implications in the understanding of mental health problems. For instance, the most important factor in the aetiology of mental distress as a result of trauma exposure is not in the events *per se*, but in the constellation of meanings and interpretations that are shaped by the cultural system of values and norms.

Another example is that the main source of mental distress of a woman who spent all her life in the war zone may not be in any way related to what happened during the war. Although she may have experienced the most terrible events in the wake of the war, her mental distress may be caused solely by the fact that she cannot give birth. Both male and female infertility, in particular among women, can lead to a social stigmatization. In cultural terms, a woman in this condition is classified as still being a child. She can never grow up and is condemned to live forever under extreme dependence on the goodwill of men. In this case, her infertility may overshadow her experiences of war exposure. Therefore, the items of the Harvard Trauma Questionnaire (HTQ) (Mollica et al., 1996) do not seem relevant to these people, even if they give positive answers to all traumatic events. Gender issues should be fully understood when trying to study the prevalence of mental disorders.

Following the examples described above, epidemiologists of mental disorders in non-Western societies may be left with empty hands. There are no available and reliable starting point instruments. In the absence of universal standardized instruments, the understanding of mental health problems requires cultural sensitivity and comprehensive approaches to develop intervention strategies in both clinical and community settings. The development of these approaches requires a great deal of time and intellectual investment. In a country such as Mozambique, characterized by ethnocultural diversity, regional socio-economic asymmetries, and a considerable degree of intellectual laziness, the field of mental health is still in its infancy and it will remain in such a position for a long period of time.

Mental distress as a disruption of sociocultural, historical and political processes

When someone suffers from a mental health problem the question of aetiology is automatically raised. There is no specification of a psychic functioning. The aetiology is intrinsically related not to a single and easily identified psychophysiological origin but to multiple complex reasons. In most of the traditional cultural systems, a disorder is at the same time psychic, somatic, familial, social, and religious (Nathan, 1999). The aetiology can range from events that occurred in the realm of the living to the realm of the dead, which in turn influences the health-seeking behaviour of the patient, accompanied by family members. The same type of reasoning is applied to the consequences of overwhelming experiences, which are explained in the first place in terms of the deregulation and disruption of sociocultural, historical and political processes (Bolton, 2001; Englund, 1998; Sideris, 2002). Post-traumatic stress syndrome (APA, 1994) is not recognized and any attempt to use such a Western type of categorization is likely to generate panic and misunderstanding among war survivors. Concepts such as 'to think', 'to remember', 'difficult to concentrate', and 'to feel alienated and detached' are very difficult to translate accurately in the local language. Time and again, although translations can be made, the people do not use these terms in their daily life.

For instance, the act of 'thinking' is seldom manifested as a cognitive process. To think is always related to an event that will take place in real life. In this way, when asking people if they sometimes think about war events, the question is perceived as if the psychologist is implying that they are planning to conduct another war. Therefore, the question is immediately rejected and they begin to distrust the psychologist. When the same question is formulated in a general way, it risks losing its meaning. For example, the first question of the Self-rating Inventory for PTSD (SIP; Hovens, 1994) is related to 'recurrent unpleasant memories'. This question was perceived as being very generic. By specifying the concept of 'past events', it has to be associated with 'war' and then the question becomes clear. However, the required specification gives rise to another problem because the concept of 'war' (locally designated by *Nkondo*) acts as a frightening stimulus.

Another constraint can arise when dealing with symptoms related to feelings. There are no linguistic distinctions between 'feeling' and 'hearing'. To feel becomes meaningful by pointing to something more concrete. Asking if a person 'feels that past events were happening again' does not make direct sense. It could only make sense if the person did experience the pain at present. Otherwise the abstraction involved in the association of feelings with past events has no consistence and the person becomes confused.

The problems presented in the two examples demonstrate that in such circumstances it is very difficult to make an accurate diagnosis and it is not possible to establish and develop a therapeutic relationship. Only through the use of a comprehensive frame of reference is it possible to define health problems from the 'emic' viewpoint. The meaningfulness of war disruptions can be observed at the sociocultural level. The manifestation of long-term war-related consequences is found through the several cases of spirit possession, mainly among young girls, which leads inevitably to family instability and depression among women. There are continual reports of cases of domestic and community violence (in particular against women), generation conflicts, reduced feelings of community belonging and identity, and a lack of confidence in the self and in the future. In addition, the long-term effects of trauma exposure were also observed in the disruption of important practices such as *Madzawde* (Igreja, 2003a), which is a child-rearing practice, and *Ntsanganiko*, which is a long and complex ceremony surrounding death and loss of a loved one. *Madzawde* is a mechanism that regulates the relationship of the child with the mother, the family in general, and the community. It is also the cultural, social and historical recognition of the vulnerabilities of the child in this particular developmental stage and the need to create a safe and protective environment that can guarantee the child's harmonious physical and psychological growth. Additionally, it is a ceremony that is performed two years after the birth of the child to release him or her from, and to close, the first stage of childhood. It is also the time of establishment of a new life cycle for the parents and the process of preparation for new offspring. When the parents fail to perform *Madzawde* or when a break occurs, then *Madzawde* turns into a set of physical symptoms that affects the child. It can lead to his or her death if treatment is not provided in time.

Ntsanganiko is also a concept used to designate a constellation of physical symptoms resulting from the breaking of this important passage ritual. In addition, people were also frustrated and desperate because of what they consider as exclusion from NGOs and government programmes.

The strategies to address such types of problems may not be understood by mental health professionals loaded with Western psychiatric knowledge. What is necessary is an in-depth understanding of the limitations and potential of local cultural resources in this post-war period. For instance, women survivors of rape, or former female soldiers, encounter many stumbling blocks to re-integrating in their community, regardless of the fact that several traditional healers have validated their experiences of suffering through the performance of different cultural therapeutic interventions. In Gorongosa, the most popular cleansing ritual is designated *Ku Patizana*. This ritual was historically applied in times of social harmony to re-establish family ties as a result of extra-marital sexual intercourse performed by either spouse. During and after the war, some traditional healers adapted *Ku Patizana* to try to help women survivors of rape or forced marriage. Although the ritual provides a cultural acknowledgement of the raped woman, it does not alleviate the psychic pain and stigmatization experienced by the rape survivors. It appears that something is 'out of tune' within traditional cultural therapies and it requires a careful and critical understanding in order to improve the quality of mental health of war survivors.

The agricultural cycle and trauma recovery

The role and importance of local resources to boost the trauma recovery process, or mental health in general, cannot be confined to the interventions developed by traditional healers, religious leaders and the customary justice system. The relationship between the agricultural cycle and trauma recovery was one of the most important findings from the research project in Gorongosa. The agricultural cycle plays a crucial and decisive role in individual and community strategies to recover from war trauma. By definition, the agricultural cycle represents a set of different periods in which there are specific activities in the fields. For each of the periods there are different levels of physical demand and involvement from the people. According to the structure and dynamics of the cycle there are periods where men and women in rural areas spend much more time in the fields in comparison with other periods during the year. These systematic changes that occur during the year have a strong influence on the psychological life of trauma survivors. As a result, there are periods of the year when trauma survivors present more distressful, intrusive symptoms than other periods. Within this context, the agricultural cycle provides a structure for daily life, and it could function as a diagnostic mechanism to separate critical cases from non-critical cases. Specifically, the agricultural cycle could help to select individuals who are susceptible to change in their symptomatology from the critical ones, i.e. those that are not affected by the positive changes registered in the social milieu.

Comprehensive and longitudinal approaches in mental health

The nature and type of aetiological theories pertaining to mental and physical health in non-Western countries requires comprehensive approaches (Das et al., 2001; Kleinman et al., 1997; Nathan, 1999). The absence of systematic studies on the quality of care provided by traditional and religious healers, together with the unavailability of professional forms of mental health care, negatively influences the psychosocial well-being of the majority of Mozambicans. The need for longitudinal approaches to carefully investigate and generate knowledge that may be instrumental for both policy development and clinical and community interventions is recognized.

We now know, better than in the past, that when someone is suffering and diagnosed with *N'Fukua*, a spirit possession, trance or dissociation state, we are not simply faced with a psycho-physiological phenomenon. Among the Gorongosas, there is a traditional belief that if someone dies in an unnatural way, particularly in the case of assassination, the spirit of the dead person sooner or later comes back to take revenge. This type of spirit is called *N'Fukua*. The revenge of *N'Fukua* is not necessarily directed against the person who committed the crime: *N'Fukua* can take revenge against any blood relative of the one who broke the natural law by killing someone else. The sole characteristic of the revenge of *N'Fukua* is to wreak havoc among the people involved in his/her assassination. Revenge is made through physical signs, such as diseases that may lead to death, and through dissociation states. Because of the diseases and uncontrolled lapses of dissociation, people consult a traditional healer. *N'Fukua* is the expression of extreme psychosocial distress and it is also a sociocultural, moral, legal and political crisis. The same holistic conceptualization and expression of illness and suffering was observed in the southern region of Mozambique (Honwana, 1998). However, recently very important developments were registered in the traditional medicine in Gorongosa through the creation of the *Gamba* spirit (Igreja, 2003b). *Gamba* is both an expression of extreme post-war suffering, and a healing potential that is rapidly spreading throughout the whole region of central Mozambique (Igreja, 2003b; Marlin, 2001). *Gamba*, as in the case of *N'Fukua*, is the spirit of an assassinated victim that comes back to the realm of the living to seek revenge and reparation. The case of *Gamba* suggests that in the post-war period, health and justice at the individual, family and community level cannot be conceived as two separate entities. A relevant observation in this regard is made by Kleinman et al. (1997) and Das et al. (2001) that the category of social suffering and recovery encompasses conditions that simultaneously involve health, welfare, and legal, moral and religious issues. There are several examples of nurses referring *N'Fukua* and *Gamba* cases to traditional and religious healers. However, although Mozambique has a National Mental Health Programme that recognizes the co-existence of other forms of healing, as described above, the referral is done in an informal and hidden manner because when discovered by their superiors, nurses can face serious trouble. There is still a huge gap between political intentions and accepted practice.

Summary

This chapter has tried to describe the situation of mental health in Mozambique, a country characterized by a plurality of medical systems and a prolonged exposure to armed violence and rapid socio-economic changes. The country is one of the very poor around the world and this condition is reflected in the state's sponsored health system. The field of professional mental health care is very limited and only a few urban people have this right in some way guaranteed. Besides the chronic lack of human and financial resources, the mental health sector has never been a priority of any government prior to or after independence.

The role of local cultural resources was never included as part of a strategy to fulfil the mental health needs of the general population. Historically, the Portuguese settlers persecuted traditional and religious healers. In the post-colonial period, the Mozambican government led by

Frelimo paradoxically continued the same policy of rejection and denial of medical pluralism. These policies represented a backward step in the process of building and developing a culturally sensitive national mental health strategy.

The consequences of the prolonged civil war on the well-being of children and the implementation of political reforms led to the creation of the first National Mental Health Programme in 1996. Within the framework of this programme, the role of local resources was publicly recognized and the establishment of partnerships between the Ministry of Health with different NGOs, including AMETRAMO, was reinforced. Unfortunately, the different governments in the post-war period hitherto were unable to develop a clear policy regarding the role and place of traditional healers. According to the political appetite of the Ministry of Health, advances were or were not made. It appears that the changes registered on the political agenda after the collapse of Marxist–Leninist policies were merely circumstantial. The changes that led to the recognition of a pluralistic society were not inspired by the intrinsic necessity to re-order society so that the different groups and cultural identities could be accommodated. Political professional debates using the discourse of 'traditional resources' are only important during electoral periods. After elections the discourse and practice of modernity replaces tradition-related vocabulary.

The majority of initiatives aimed at providing mental health services for the poor populations, particularly survivors of violence, have been led by NGOs in partnership with international organizations. However, lack of financial resources and culturally sensitive knowledge represents the main stumbling block in the provision of more humane and decent care.

References

American Psychiatric Association (1994) Diagnostic and Statistical Manual of Mental Disorders. (4th edition) Washington, DC: APA.

Bolton P (2001) Local perceptions of the mental health effects of the Rwandan Genocide. Journal of Nervous and Mental Disease, 189(4): 243–8.

Bondestam S (1994) Mental health. In Lankinen K, Bergstrom S, Makela P, Peltomaa M (Eds.) Health and Disease in Developing Countries. London and Basingstoke: Macmillan.

Bracken P, Giller J, Summerfield D (1995) Psychological responses of war and atrocity: Limitations of current concepts. Social Science and Medicine, 40(8): 1073–82.

Das V, Kleinman A, Lock M, Ramphele M, Reynolds P (2001) Remaking a world: Violence, social suffering, and recovery. Berkeley: University of California Press.

Eisenbruch M (1991) From post-traumatic stress disorder to cultural bereavement: Diagnosis of Southeast Asian refugees. Social Science and Medicine, 33(6): 673–80.

Englund H (1998) Death, trauma, and ritual: Mozambican refugees in Malawi. Social Science and Medicine, 46: 1165–74.

German G (1987) Mental health in Africa: The extent of mental health problems in Africa today. An update of epidemiological knowledge. British Journal of Psychiatry, 151: 435–9.

Green E (1996) Indigenous Healers and the African State: Policy Issues Concerning African Indigenous Healers in Mozambique and Southern Africa. United Nations Plaza, New York: Pact Publications.

Hiegel J (1994) Use of indigenous concepts and healers in the care of refugees: Some experiences from the Thai border camps. In Marsella A, Bornemann T, Ekblad S, Orley J (Eds.) Amidst Peril and Pain: The Mental Health of and Well Being of the World's Refugees. Washington, DC: American Psychological Association. pp. 293–309.

Honwana A (1998) Sealing the past, facing the future: Trauma healing in rural Mozambique. In Accord, Issue no. 3. London: Conciliation Resources.

Hovens J (1994) Research into Psychodynamic of Posttraumatic Stress Disorder. The Netherlands: Eburon Press.

Igreja V (2003a) The effects of traumatic experiences on the infant–mother relationship in the former war-zones of central Mozambique: The case of Madzawde in Gorongosa. Infant Mental Health Journal, 24: 5.

Igreja V (2003b) Why are there many drums playing until the dawn? Exploring the role of Gamba spirits and healers in the post-war recovery period in Gorongosa, central Mozambique. Journal of Transcultural Psychiatry. In press.

Igreja V, Schreuder B, Kleijn W (1999) The cultural dimension of war traumas in central Mozambique: The case of Gorongosa. Transcultural Mental Health On-Line, pp. 1–13. www.priory.com/psych/traumacult.htm

Kleinman A, Das V, Lock M (1997) Social Suffering. Berkeley: University of California Press.

Mandlhate C (1996) Programmea nacional de saúde mental. Ministério da Saúde. Direcção Nacional de Saúde. Secção de Saúde Mental. Maputo. [National Mental Health Programme.]

Marlin R (2001) Possessing the past: Legacies of violence and reproductive illness in central Mozambique. PhD dissertation. New Brunswick: State University of New Jersey.

Marsella A, Friedman MJ, Gerrity ET, Scurfield RM (1996) Ethnocultural Aspects of PTSD: Issues, Research, and Clinical Applications. Washington, DC: American Psychological Association.

Mollica R, Caspi-Yavin Y, Lavelle J, Tor S, Yang T, Chan S, Pham T, Ryan A, De Marneffe D (1996) The Harvard Trauma Questionnaire (HTQ) Manual: Cambodian, Laotian and Vietnamese Versions. Cambridge, MA: Harvard School of Public Health.

Nathan T (1999) Le sperme du diable: Éléments d'ethnopsychotherapie. Paris: Presses Universitaires de France.

Schreuder B, Igreja V, van Dijk J, Kleijn W (2001) Intrusive re-experiencing of chronic strife or war. Advances in Psychiatric Treatment, 7: 102–8.

Sideris T (2002) War, gender and culture: Mozambican women refugees. Social Science and Medicine. In press.

United Nations Development Programme (1999) Mozambique. Economic growth and human development: Progress, obstacles and challenges. UNDP, Maputo – Mozambique.

World Health Organization (1997) Intercountry Workshop on Community Based Psychosocial Rehabilitation in Post-Armed Conflict Countries. Maputo, 27–30 October.

World Health Organization (2000) Second Intercountry Workshop on Community Based Psychosocial Rehabilitation in Post-Armed Conflict Countries. Harare, 21–23 March.

CHAPTER ELEVEN

Conclusion

PETER MORRALL AND MIKE HAZELTON

The widespread acknowledgement that mental health is an important human rights concern has coincided with recognition that the global cost of mental illness is considerable. Nevertheless, as the case studies presented throughout this book attest, it is by no means a straightforward matter to respond effectively to the problem of human rights in mental health policy and practice. In developed countries, between 7% and 14% of national budgets are typically allocated to health, with a reasonable proportion of this going to mental health. In developing countries, this figure is much more likely to be in the order of 1% to 5%, and in some cases mental health is virtually overlooked. However, the experience of developed countries suggests that wide-ranging policy developments, including substantial additional funding for mental health services do not necessarily translate into a better quality of life for those with mental illness.

While it can be demonstrated that hospital bed populations have declined, that hospitals have been closed, and that new, more comprehensive services have been developed, it is more difficult to show that there has been a reduction in discrimination related to mental illness; or that community knowledge of disorders such as depression and schizophrenia has improved; or that those who suffer from mental health problems and disorders are now better able to live in the community with the full range of entitlements of citizenship. Moreover, the extent to which it might be possible to improve the life circumstances and safeguard the human rights of the mentally ill depends on more than the living situation, social support and occupational opportunity provided by health and human services. Much also depends on the attitudes of the staff providing the services, and on public opinion (Hazelton and Clinton, 2002: 99), and it has been suggested that even in liberal-democratic countries, such as the UK, the limits of public tolerance for mentally ill people living in the community may already have been reached (Campbell, 1999).

In the UK the development of post-liberal mental health policies and legislation has been associated with intense media and public concern over the 'shortcomings' of psychiatric services and the 'threat' to public order posed by unsupervised mentally ill people in the community (Morrall 2000, 2002). In a political climate overly sensitive to law and order concerns, and attuned to the 'failures' of the mental health system, there is a risk of the psychiatric professions adopting defensive postures, and the concerns of service users being drowned out in the general din of allegation and denial (Laurance, 2003). Under such circumstances it is difficult to imagine policy-making being clear-minded or strategic, or how human rights concerns might be addressed in a sensitive and balanced manner.

As the chapter outlining recent health care system changes in the USA illustrates, developments in health economics and governance are also influencing mental health policies and practices in important ways. In the case of the USA, the boundary between clinical judgement and administrative expectation is being redrawn, and increasingly autonomous and discretionary decision-making by clinical service providers is being subjected to the influence of health managers. However, it is important to question whether the focus on changing the balance between clinical judgement and administrative expectation may be distracting policymakers and health professionals from the most important consideration – improving the quality of life of service users.

The experience of mental health reform in Australia illustrates the difficulties of translating policies into improvements in the lives of service users. While a decade-long programme of reforms has resulted in increased budgets and improved services, progress in combating discrimination and upholding the human rights of the mentally ill has been uneven and slow. Many health professionals continue to display poor attitudes towards the mentally ill, and the inadequate provision of community services such as rehabilitation, housing, employment and community support has left many service users seriously under-supported in the community. When evaluated in terms of whether or not those with mental illness are now better able to live as citizens in the community, the success of the National Mental Health Strategy (Australian Health Ministers, 1992) has been very limited.

With its origins in controversial reforms advocating the closure of psychiatric hospitals, the mental health reforms in Italy have resulted in what is possibly the most comprehensive and disseminated network of community psychiatric services in the world. While building up services in the community took time, the Italian experience suggests that community care can meet the mental health needs of a population, including those with the most severe disorders. The generally relaxed and collaborative relationship that Italian mental health consumer and carer organizations have with mental health services suggests a community-based mental health system that is largely meeting the needs of its clientele, and is sensitive to the types of human rights concerns that remain controversial in so many other countries.

If there are mixed reports on mental health and human rights in developed countries, the situation in many developing countries ranges from struggling to very serious. In the case of Egypt we find relatively well-developed psychiatric services, and long-standing mental health legislation. While reform priorities suggest the influence of Western policy directions, traditional and religious healers also have an important role, especially in providing primary psychiatric care. However, there is the issue, also likely to be found in other countries, of psychiatric professionals with Western-styled training finding themselves at odds with public sentiment when dealing with clients whose behaviour (e.g. homosexuality) violates traditional and religious norms. Paradoxically, a psychiatric diagnosis may sometimes provide the only escape from the stigma and punishment associated with a serious social and religious transgression.

Policymakers in India are undertaking mental health reforms in a developing country with a massive population, meagre infrastructure and an insufficient number of health professionals. Under the conditions of limited government investment in health, widespread poverty, and low rates of literacy, community care has necessarily meant care *by* the community rather than care *in* the community. Ensuring minimum standards of mental health care for the population, increasing the mental health-related skill level of the primary care health workforce, and increasing mental health literacy and community participation in the development of mental health services have been the main reform priorities. While progress in implementing mental health programmes has been slow, the tragedy in Erwadi in late 2001 has focused public and media attention on the human rights of the mentally ill, and accelerated the pace of reform.

Brazil provides a fascinating instance of nation-building incorporating re-democratization following the end of military dictatorship. In the last two decades, Brazilian mental health services, along with other human services, have undergone sweeping changes. Beginning with a process of humanization and re-democratization which commenced with the end of the military dictatorship in the 1980s, the reforms have now progressed to the point where a communitarian mental health system is being implemented. The implementation of a new system of psychosocial treatment centres has coincided with a planned reduction in psychiatric hospital beds. At the heart of the reforms has been a broad orientation towards community participation, which pervades Brazilian politics, from the municipal through to the national level. That mental health has been embraced as a key element of this democratizing trend in public policy is both a model for, and a powerful statement to, the international community.

We noted in the Introduction how despotic regimes of both the left and the right have used psychiatry as an instrument of social oppression. While different in important ways, the cases of post-Soviet Russia and the People's Republic of China illustrate how the misuse of psychiatry for political purposes continues into the present.

There is a long history of psychiatry being used to control dissident populations in Russia, both in Tsarist and Soviet times. Following the collapse of the Soviet Union and a brief period of democratization and normalization within psychiatric services, mental health policy and practice is again being shaped by the priorities of the state in the Russian Federation. The war in Chechnya has resulted in a political climate in which the development of public policy, including mental health policy, has stagnated. There is no co-ordinated response to serious problems such as alcohol abuse and suicide, and it is unlikely that these problems can be satisfactorily addressed without the widespread involvement of society. While the reform process has slowed, it nonetheless continues, especially in regional areas. To date, however, there is little evidence of mental health being seen as a priority in Russian public policy.

The campaign of persecution and terror which the government of the People's Republic of China has directed towards the practitioners of Falun Gong represents a gross misuse of psychiatry for state political purposes, with many mental health facilities and professionals being drawn into the use of persecution, torture and even murder. This startling instance of the abuse of psychiatry leading to gross human rights violations, including unnecessary psychiatric treatment, imprisonment, and torture, is testimony that psychiatry remains vulnerable to exploitation by the state in countries governed by authoritarian political regimes. It remains to be seen whether the recent change in party leadership and the weight of international condemnation will see an end to the serious human rights abuses perpetrated on those identified with Falun Gong.

Finally, there are countries for which establishing even the most essential level of mental health care is a human rights issue. With a history of colonial exploitation, post-colonial armed conflict, poverty and famine, Mozambique provides a stark lesson in the challenges faced by very poor countries in providing basic standards of health and well-being for the population. Despite the trauma of war, poverty and famine, and with the vast majority of the population having no access to health professionals, mental health has never been a priority in Mozambique. Moreover, the colonial policy of persecuting traditional and religious healers was continued during the period of Communist government, and more recently, successive governments have largely ignored the contribution that these traditional practitioners might make to mental health care. Given the severely limited opportunities for human development, the inclusion of religious and cultural practices in primary care could provide for the needs of the majority of Mozambicans, who have virtually no other means of dealing with mental health problems.

Throughout both the developed and the developing areas of the world, mental health has undoubtedly entered the political domain. In recent decades governments in many countries have moved to implement policies through which to co-ordinate and direct the development of mental health services. As the case studies presented throughout this book indicate, while these policies reflect local circumstances and requirements, they also exhibit a number of similar concerns, such as commitment to service development, continuous quality improvement, service accountability, cost-effectiveness, mainstreaming mental health services within the general health sector, and sensitivity to human rights.

Mental health reform is never a straightforward matter, but budgets can be shown to have increased and improvements in services can be measured. However, while documents and statements of human rights exist, this in no way guarantees their implementation in practice (Watchirs, 2000). Underpinning projects to ensure the human rights of those with mental illness are economic policies, social change, political will and especially public attitudes. All of these factors may facilitate or impede the implementation of human rights provisions.

In the field of mental health, as in other areas of human development, safeguarding and extending human rights involves political contestation. While democracy may well be a precondition of human rights, there is no guarantee that these will not be eroded or revoked, even under the conditions of liberal democracy. Moreover, the mobilization of the USA and its 'new world order' collaborators, while ostensibly promulgating democracy and human rights (to the point of armed conflict, for example, in Afghanistan and Iraq), undermines established international mechanisms and institutions promoting justice and representative governance. If the future is to be one in which the human rights of the mentally ill are to be safeguarded, this will require ongoing vigilance and activism within the context of this new world order.

References

Australian Health Ministers (1992) National Mental Health Policy, Canberra: Australian Government Publishing Service.

Campbell P (1999) The consumer of mental health care. In Newell R, Gourney K (Eds.) Mental Health Nursing: An Evidence-Based Approach. Edinburgh: Churchill-Livingstone. pp. 11–26.

Hazelton M, Clinton M (2002) Mental health consumers or citizens with mental health problems? In Henderson S, Petersen A (Eds.) Consuming Health: The Commodification of Health Care. London: Routledge. pp. 88–101.

Laurance J (2003) Pure Madness: How Fear Drives the Mental Health System. London: Routledge.

Morrall PA (2000) Madness and Murder. London: Whurr.

Morrall PA (2002) Madness, murder, and social control. Mental Health Today. August: 23–5.

Watchirs H (2000) Application of rights analysis instrument to Australian mental health legislation. Report to the Australian Health Ministers' Advisory Council National Mental Health Working Group. Canberra: Commonwealth Department of Health and Aged Care.

Index